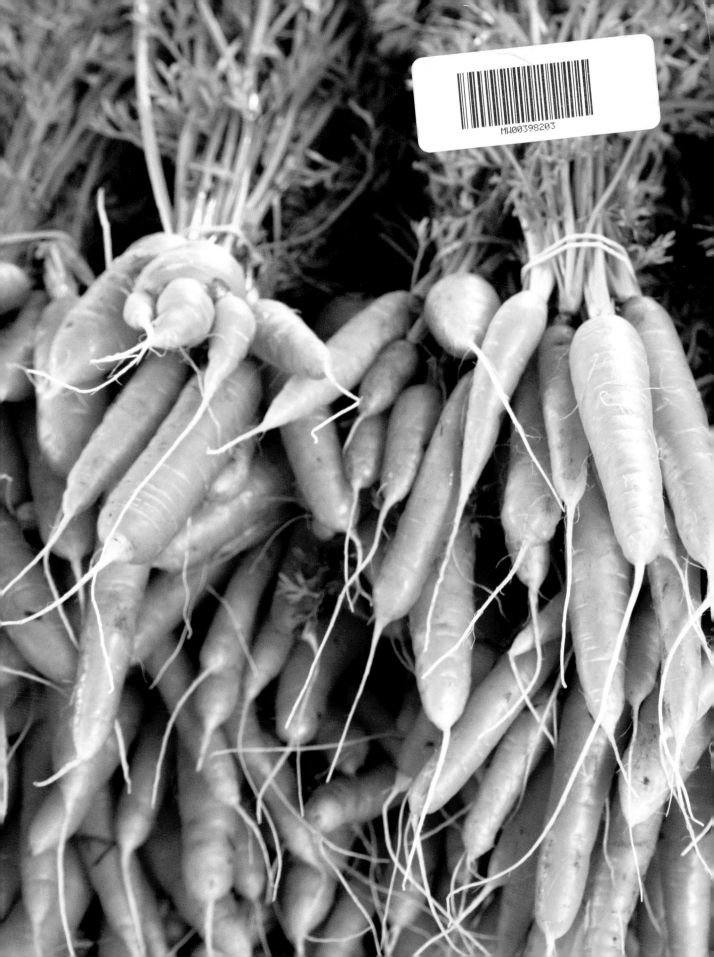

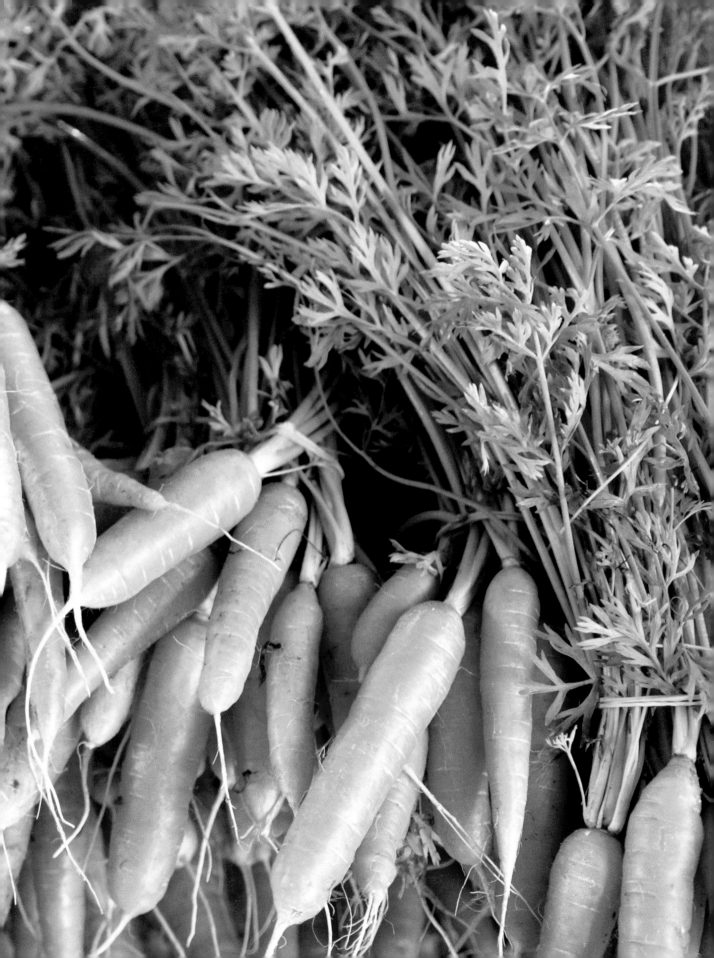

VISIONARY KITCHEN

A COOKBOOK FOR EYE HEALTH

Live Well,
Eat Well,
See Well —
Sandra a Young, OD

SANDRA YOUNG, OD

PHOTOGRAPHS BY ANNE MARIE COUTTS, DTR

Library of Congress Control Number: 2013949934
ISBN 978-0-615-86697-0

Edited by Sandra Young, OD and John Casbon, MD
Nutritional Analysis by Anne Marie Coutts, SELF Nutrition
Photography & Food Styling by Anne Marie Coutts • am.coutts@gmail.com
Designed by Russell Sadeghpour • russell.sadeghpour@gmail.com

To place an order, please visit www.visionarykitchen.com
or call (800) 688-6815

Favorite Recipe Press
An imprint of Southwestern Publishing Group, Inc.
P.O. Box 305142
Nashville, TN 37230
(800) 358-0560

On the front cover: Striped Bass with Mediterranean Tapenade (page 128)
On the back cover: Bison Chili (page 102), Almond Macaroons (page 211)

Disclaimer
The recipes in this book were created using ingredients with nutrients thought to support ocular health. No claim is made that consumption of these foods or recipes will improve vision, ocular disease or ocular health. This book is not intended to diagnose, treat, cure or prevent any disease. Before beginning any new diet plan, first consult with your physician. While this book was developed with ocular health in mind, consumption of these foods or recipes will not replace regular eye health examinations by a qualified optometrist or ophthalmologist.

Vision is a precious gift.

This book is dedicated to those with a desire
to eat and cook more healthfully.

Live Well, Eat Well, See Well!

Writing a book requires a dedicated team;
writing a cookbook requires a dedicated team with dishpan hands!

I want to thank Anne Marie Coutts, my tireless photographer, nutritionist and niece!

I wonder how many cookbook authors have a triple board certified physician as their sous chef? Thank you Jon M. Casbon, MD, MPH (Col., USAF, Retired) for your help in the test kitchen, your advice and editing skills.

Thank you to Judy Halter, my friend and food stylist, for all your help and support. Your artistic flair helped to create beautiful table scapes.

The graphic design is unparalleled in this book. Awesome job, Russell Sadeghpour. Thank you!

I want to thank Kathy Villere and Marianne Hastings for their contributions. It's amazing how many eyes its takes to see all the details to create a quality book.

Thank you Ellen Troyer, MT, MA, my mentor and friend, you have believed in me and my book from the start.

Thank you to my husband, Michael E. Young, OD, FAAO (Col., USAF, Retired) chief taste tester and ocular nutrition advisor. Your love and moral support has made this cookbook possible.

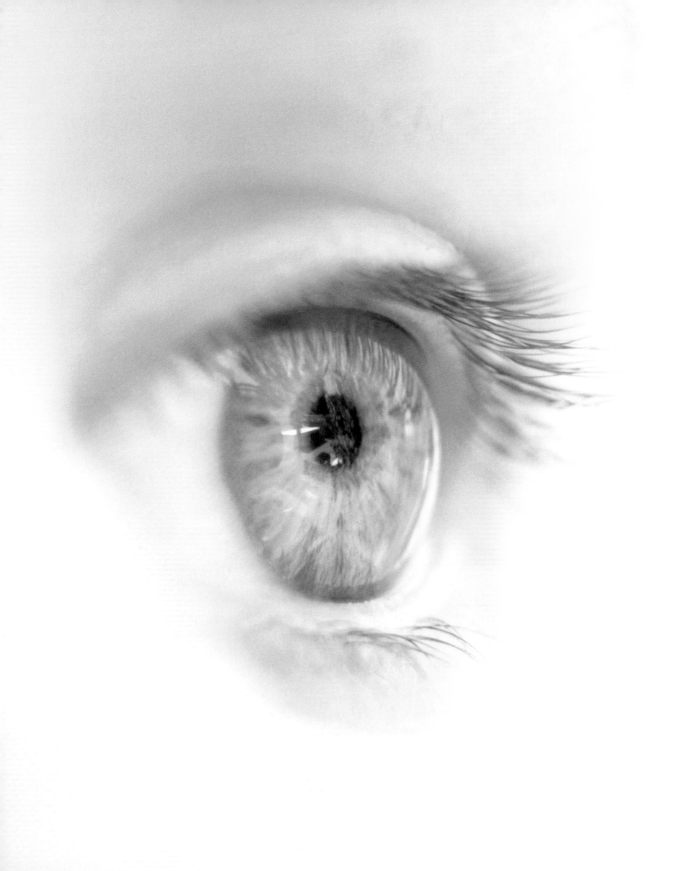

CONTENTS

FOREWORD BY ELLEN TROYER

Major Kudos to Sandra Young, OD for writing a much needed cookbook focused on ocular health. When we are extraordinarily lucky, nutrient-dense healthy food is one of our most accessible pleasures. It's more of an art than a science and truly belongs in the realm of the senses. Great recipes are born from natural ingredient knowledge, instinct, and a vivid imagination. Visionary Kitchen suggests that Dr. Young is blessed with all three.

LIVING WELL AND STAYING HEALTHY IN TODAY'S BRAVE NEW WORLD

Most of us lead busy lives and many of us too often think we don't have time to cook from scratch. We resort to chemically-altered and overly-processed fast foods, or prepared super market foods now scientifically linked to increased risk of illness and obesity. Developing instincts about natural foods and spices is worth cultivating. I promise you will have fun while doing so, and will be healthier and happier for the effort.

WOW MOMENTS

Dr. Sandra Young's recipes are culinary road maps to nutrient-dense fine dining. The ingredients in her recipes link brain to stomach naturally. Speaking as an artistic science person, extraordinary flavor affinities actually do exist, and when they happen, it's like throwing a switch in the brain -- we just know it. At that moment, the harmonic convergence of food and flavorings become so exceptional that we are transported into some other world of unreal flavor sensations. So be careful. WOW moments such as these can be addictive. Fine nutrient-dense food lovers are powerless to resist them; intrigued to pursue them, or at least have great fun trying.

SHE'S THE HEALTHY SPICE QUEEN

Sandra Young is fearless where spices are concerned and her recipes prove she has mastered the art of incorporating different and unusual spices into her original recipes or redesigned classic recipes to add vital nutrients, while enhancing natural ingredient flavors instead of overpowering them. She understands that food can take us on an adventure without leaving our homes. Her recipes are a healthy culinary trip around the world in far more than 80 days if you choose to try them all. She introduces us to nutrient-dense North American, South American, Asian, Indian, Italian, French, Turkish, Greek and many other country's dishes that promise to delight your family and friends palates while adding to their micronutrient intake.

MORE PLEASURE: LESS DENIAL

Sandy's recipes prove that beautifully presented nutrient-dense foods nurture body and soul and should be viewed as our primary source of nutrition. She speaks to the health and economic needs of the present, which requires that we take more personal responsibility for preventing diseases instead of being dependent on modern medicine and pharmacology to treat issues that we can prevent with healthier lifestyles. Disease treatments are not nearly as much fun and are proving to be economically unsustainable for us individually and for our country. We must commit to making healthier lifestyle choices, including the foods we eat, the exercise we get, and the passions we choose if we expect to live long energetic lives filled with joy.

Ellen Troyer, MT MA
Biosyntrx CEO / Chief Research Officer

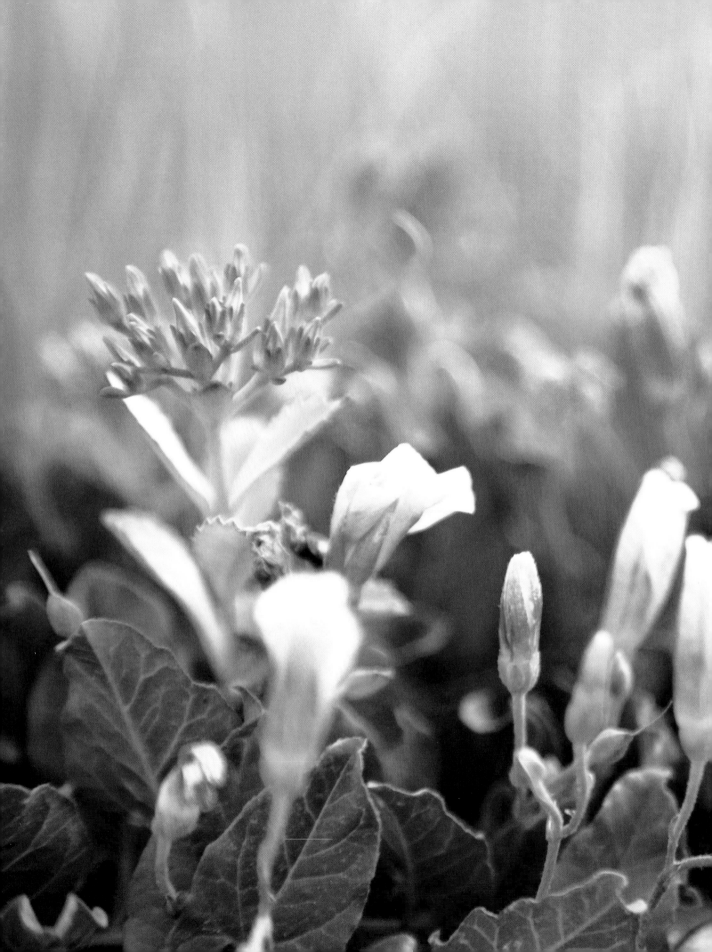

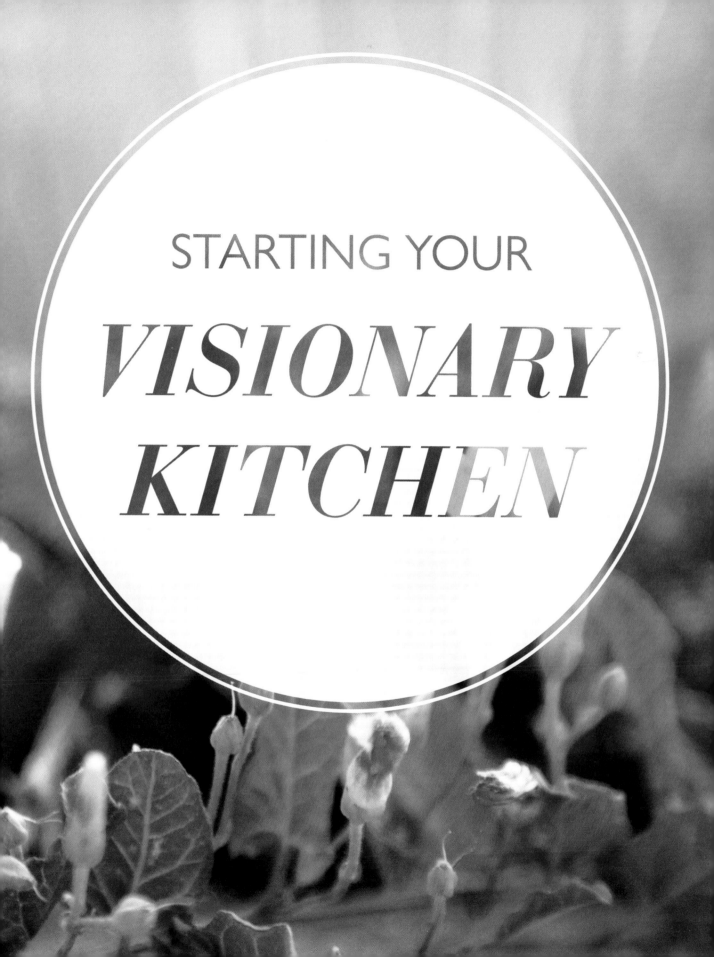

STARTING YOUR

VISIONARY

KITCHEN

Each of the recipes,
as well as the cooking
techniques presented in
Visionary Kitchen:
A Cookbook for Eye Health
are carefully designed to
support optimal ocular
health and vision.

WELCOME TO THE

VISIONARY KITCHEN

Whole foods have a symphony of nutrients working together in concert to provide the potential for optimal health and well being. Recent studies have highlighted the importance of several individual nutrients that support eye health. All the recipes in *Visionary Kitchen* use these eye nutrients to create tasty and healthful dishes.

For quick reference, this book includes lists of foods loaded with specific nutrients needed to maximize eye health potential. In order for the body to utilize as many of these nutrients as possible, food preparation and food combinations are important. Excess heat and lengthy cooking times diminish the vitamin content in foods. Lightly sautéing or pureeing kale or spinach will break down the plant cell structure to give the body more access to the nutrients present. The fat soluble nutrients, lutein+zeaxanthin, can be more easily absorbed by the body when eaten with a small amount of healthy fat.

Special attention has been given to herbs and spices, not only because they make food taste great, but also because they are nutritional powerhouses. Fresh or dried herbs and spices have wonderful health benefits for the eyes and body.

This cookbook is written for a variety of dietary requirements and choices, including gluten-free, vegan, vegetarian, dairy-free and meat-eaters alike. There are recipes for large holiday gatherings, single serving meals before work, as well as snacks and meals on-the-go. Every day can be an eye and vision health day!

Each recipe features a short list of important "eye nutrients." Amounts are listed per serving.

Lycopene • 3,474mcg
Omega-3 • 1,237mg
Vitamin C • 69%DV

For full nutritional analysis of all recipes please visit
www.visionarykitchen.com

EYE HEALTH, VISION & NUTRITION

Through a combination of important micronutrients and essential fatty acids, proper blood sugar regulation and attentive cooking techniques, eye health can be promoted through everyday nutrition.

The key nutrients listed in this chapter comprise the cornerstones of the recipes in this book.

The eyes are highly metabolically active and have unique nutritional needs. Recent science has identified some of the key nutrients for optimal eye health, including:

- Lutein+Zeaxanthin
- Omega-3 fatty acids
  balanced with Omega-6 fatty acids
- Vitamin A family
- Vitamin C
- Vitamin E
- Zinc

Regulation of blood glucose levels is also important. There are a number of other nutrients that play a role in eye health, including the B vitamins, selenium and other plant-based antioxidants.

Vision, the ability to see, is very complex. Light enters the eye and is focused on the retina. The retina converts this light information into bioelectrical signals that are then sent to the brain and interpreted as vision. If light is not properly focused on the retina, glasses, contact lenses or refractive surgery can be used to correct the focus. An out-of-focus eye can be a healthy eye. Healthy eyes may need glasses or contacts to correct eye sight to 20/20. However, even an unhealthy eye may retain 20/20 sight. Healthy eyes and excellent vision should be enjoyed for a lifetime. The nutrients emphasized in *Visionary Kitchen* are directed at supporting the health and well being of ocular tissues. The following pages discuss nutrient information and their food sources.

ESSENTIAL MICRONUTRIENTS

*VITAMIN A FAMILY > CAROTENOIDS >
XANTHOPHYLLS > LUTEIN + ZEAXANTHIN*

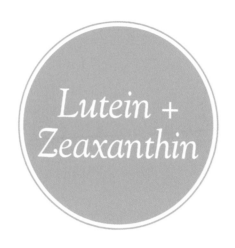

*Lutein +
Zeaxanthin*

The vitamin A found in plant sources includes over 600 carotenoids. Of importance to the eye are two subclasses of carotenoids known as the carotenes and xanthophylls. The xanthophylls lutein and zeaxanthin are two carotenoids known to be present in the crystalline lens and retina of the eye. These essential pigments help to reduce oxidative stress and absorb blue and UV light offering protection to the lens and macula from their harmful effects.

A diet rich in these nutrients can help ensure sensitive structures within the eye remain healthy. In particular, the lutein and zeaxanthin found in egg yolks is highly bioavailable and preferentially accumulates in the macular region of the retina.

Food Sources of Lutein+Zeaxanthin

Egg Yolk • Goji Berries • Corn (Maize)
Olives • Zucchini • Orange Bell Pepper
Honeydew Melon • Red & Green Grapes
Orange Juice & Oranges • Cucumber • Mango
Nectarine • Peach • Tomato Juice • Green Beans
Scallion • Brussels Sprouts • Celery • Parsley
Green Peppers • Cayenne Pepper

Food Sources of Lutein

Butternut Squash • Spinach • Pumpkin • Kale
Red Delicious Apple • Tomato • Swiss Chard
Collard Greens • Kiwi • Yellow Squash • Broccoli
Peas • Romaine and Green Lettuce
Yellow Bell Pepper • Red Bell Pepper

The amount of lutein+zeaxanthin contained in a specific food is usually quantified together. The foods listed under lutein contain very little or no zeaxanthin.

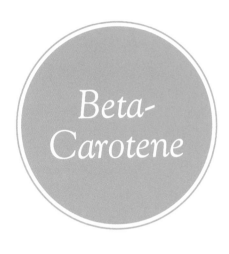

The antioxidant pigment beta-carotene gives carrots and sweet potatoes their orange color. Beta-carotene converts to vitamin A retinol in a self-limiting manner when liver stores of vitamin A are depleted. Taking beta-carotene in supplement form is not recommended because it decreases the amount of lutein and zeaxanthin transported to the eye and may increase the risk of lung cancer in smokers and former smokers. Decreased transport of lutein+zeaxanthin may decrease the density of these protective pigments in the macula. However, getting vitamin A in the diet is considered safe. Vitamin A also plays an important role in the production and stability of the tear film.

Food Sources of Beta-Carotene

Sweet Potato • Spinach • Kale • Collard Greens • Carrots • Turnip Greens • Mustard Greens
Swiss Chard • Butternut Squash • Basil • Parsley • Marjoram • Oregano • Sage • Coriander • Thyme
Red Leaf Lettuce • Cantaloupe • Green Peppers • Broccoli • Asparagus • Papaya • Red Delicious Apple
Mango • Peach • Nectarine • Dried Apricot • Honeydew • Orange Bell Pepper • Spinach • Pumpkin
Red & Green Grapes • Oranges • Winter Squash • Romaine Lettuce

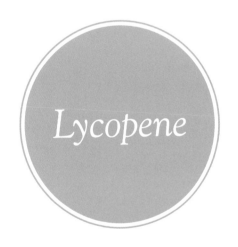

The antioxidant lycopene is responsible for giving many fruits and vegetables their red color. While many vitamins may diminish or degrade with cooking, lycopene becomes more bioavailable. Cooked tomatoes have more bioavailable lycopene than fresh tomatoes.

Lycopene helps maintain or protect the integrity of cell membranes. The antioxidant properties of lycopene may help counteract the formation of cataracts.

Food Sources of Lycopene

Sun Dried Tomato • Tomato Juice • Fresh Tomato • Cooked Tomato (*Paste, Puree, Sauce*)
Scallions • Pink and Red Grapefruit • Dried Herbs • Dried Parsley • Dried Basil • Guava
Watermelon • Asparagus • Chili Powder • Red Cabbage • Rose Hips • Papaya
Red Delicious Apples • Oranges • Persimmon • Red Bell Peppers

ESSENTIAL MICRONUTRIENTS

VITAMIN A FAMILY > RETINOIDS > RETINOL

Retinol is essential for wound healing and immune function. Preformed vitamin A, known as the retinoids retinol and retinal, is found in animal food sources. Retinol is required for the production of rhodopsin, the visual pigment used to see in low light levels. An early symptom of vitamin A deficiency is night blindness from damage to the retina. This condition is most commonly found in malnourished children in developing countries.

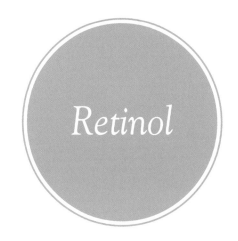

Food Sources of Retinol

Butter • Egg Yolk • Cream Cheese • Sardines • Edam Cheese • Parmesan Cheese
Mackerel • Liverwurst Chicken Liver • Duck, Veal, Goose & Turkey Liver
Liver Pâté • Cod Liver Oil

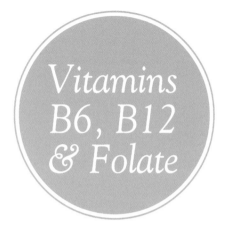

The B vitamins are a group of eight water soluble vitamins known as the B-complex. These vitamins help break down carbohydrates, fat and protein for optimal metabolism of food.

Food Sources of Vitamin B6

Garlic • Paprika • Dark Leafy Green Vegetables
Cabbage • Crimini Mushrooms • Cod • Tuna
Salmon • Broccoli • Turmeric • Liver • Turkey
Leeks

Food Sources of Vitamin B12

Liver • Clams • Mussels • Oysters • Caviar
Mackerel • Herring • Salmon • Sardines
Grass-Fed Beef • Parmesan • Feta • Egg Yolk
Shrimp • Scallops • Tofu • Miso • Sea Vegetables

Food Sources of Folate

Lentils • Chickpeas • Avocado • Romaine Lettuce
Spinach • Broccoli • Papaya • Cauliflower
Turnip Greens • Beets • Asparagus • Liver

Food Combinations with B6, B12 & Folate

Recent published research suggests vitamins B6, B12 and folate may protect women against age-related macular degeneration (AMD).

**Broccoli • Garlic • Salmon
Asparagus • Eggs • Paprika
Spinach • Garlic • Mussels**

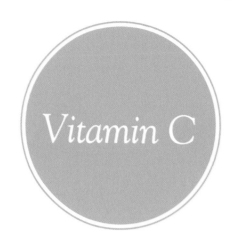

Vitamin C is a powerful, water-soluble antioxidant. Vitamin C supports wound healing and the formation of collagen, as well as protects against environmental toxins. The Age-Related Eye Disease Study (AREDS1) found that vitamin C plus beta-carotene, vitamin E and zinc slowed the progression of advanced Age-related Macular Degeneration by 25%. The amount of vitamin C contained in food decreases with cooking. Consider adding a fresh source of vitamin C to your meal by garnishing with chopped parsley.

Food Sources of Vitamin C

Red and Green Chili Pepper • Guava • Bell Pepper
Broccoli • Cauliflower • Brussels Sprouts • Kiwi • Papaya • All Citrus • Strawberries
Fresh Herbs (*Thyme, Parsley*) • Dark Leafy Greens (*Kale, Mustard Greens, Swiss Chard*)
Red Cabbage • Sun Dried Tomato • Raspberries • Celery • Pineapple • Summer Squash
Dried Herbs (*Coriander, Rosemary, Basil, Cloves, Saffron, Cayenne Pepper*)
Cantaloupe • Mango • Fresh Tomato • Chives

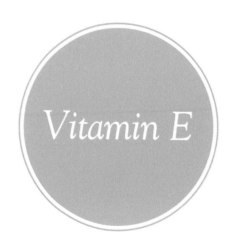

Vitamin E is a family of 8 fat soluble antioxidants, 4 tocopherols and 4 tocotrienols. Most foods contain differing levels of each form of vitamin E, with the exception of annatto seeds (achiote seeds), which have very high levels of tocotrienols. Vitamin E appears to have cardioprotective benefits as well as boosting the immune system when combined with vitamin C. Vitamin E, along with lutein and zeaxanthin from food and supplements, may decrease the risk of cataracts.

Food Sources of Vitamin E

Sunflower Seeds • Paprika • Red Chili Powder • Almonds • Pine Nuts
Peanuts • Kale • Swiss Chard • Bell Pepper • Brussels Sprouts • Wheat Germ Oil
Flax Seed Oil • Dried Apricots • Green Olives • Spinach • Kiwi • Blueberries
Herbs and Spices (*Dried Basil, Dried Oregano, Sage, Thyme, Parsley, Cumin*) • Broccoli
Tomato • Achiote Seeds • Asparagus • Butternut Squash

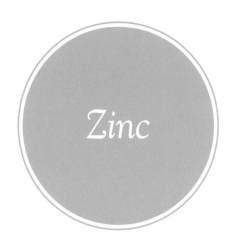

Zinc is a trace mineral involved in gene expression, immune function and cell growth. In the eye, a high concentration of zinc is found in the macula. Zinc is part of the antioxidant supplement formulation in the AREDS1 study, shown to decrease the risk of progression of macular degeneration (AMD) from the intermediate to the advanced form.

Food Sources of Zinc

Oysters • Wheat Germ • Liver • Roast Beef • Pepita Seeds • Squash Seeds
Dark Chocolate • Natural Cocoa Powder • Lamb • Peanuts • Alaskan King Crab
Sesame Seeds • Almonds • Egg Yolks • Crimini Mushrooms • Summer Squash
Asparagus • Venison • Swiss Chard • Shrimp • Collard Greens • Yogurt • Green Peas
Cashews • Chickpeas • Parsley • Anise Seed

ESSENTIAL FATTY ACIDS

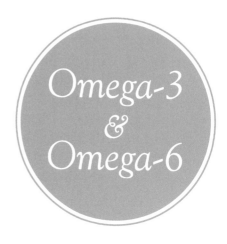

Omega-3 & Omega-6

Essential fatty acids are fatty acids which must be acquired through diet and are necessary for good health. The human body lacks the enzymes required to synthesize these polyunsaturated fatty acids.

Two essential fatty acids include omega-3 and omega-6 fatty acids. While both are important for vision, the ratio of omega-3 to omega-6 is also important. The current recommendation is a ratio of one omega-3 fatty acid to four omega-6 fatty acids. Overly processed foods, especially fried "fast foods" provide excessive omega-6 linoleic acid (LA) without the vitamin and mineral co-factors required for proper enzymatic, omega-6 metabolism, causing an imbalance between omega-3 and omega-6 fatty acids. The food sources of omega-6 fatty acids are primarily commercially sold oils including corn, peanut, soybean, grapeseed, safflower and cottonseed oils. Olive oil is the best choice for daily consumption since it has lower amounts of omega-6 fatty acids.

Both omega-3 and omega-6 essential fatty acids along with appropriate vitamin, mineral and other nutrient co-factors are required for optimal three layer tear film production. This is important in preventing or ameliorating dry eye problems.

There are three types of essential omega-3 fatty acids:

- ALA (Alpha-linolenic acid)
- EPA (Eicosapentaenoic acid)
- DHA (Docosahexaenoic acid)

Alpha linolenic acid (ALA) is found in plant sources, like flax seed. ALA helps to support cardiovascular well being. The body inefficiently converts ALA to DHA/EPA.

The omega-3 fatty acids eicosapentaenoic acid (EPA) and docosahexaenoic acid (DHA) are found together primarily in fish and fish oil. EPA is an anti-inflammatory molecule which blocks one of the enzyme pathways (delta- 5) required for a pro-inflammatory response. DHA is metabolized from EPA and its primary job is to keep cellular membranes pliable so that nutrients can enter cells and metabolic waste materials can exit cells. This is particularly important for eye and brain health.

Omega-6 fatty acids help to produce an appropriate lifesaving, pro-inflammatory effect when needed. Examples of this include: swelling to protect a broken bone, a fever spike to kill off bacteria and viruses, and clotting when bleeding.

Food Sources of EPA/DHA Omega-3

Salmon (*Wild, Canned, Smoked, Sockeye, King, Coho*) • Herring • Mackerel • Whitefish Anchovies • Sardines • Rainbow Trout Arctic Char • Caviar • Tilapia • Striped Bass Mussels • Squid (*Calamari*) • Sole • Flounder Dungeness Crab • Shrimp • Scallops Catfish • Oysters • Clams • Haddock • Cod Cray Fish • Mahi-Mahi • Lobster • Bluefish Wild Grouper • Wild Sea Bass • Albacore Yellow Fin Tuna • Halibut

Food Sources of ALA Omega-3

Tofu • Soy Beans • Spirulina • Seaweed Flax Seeds • Butternut Squash Seeds • Chia Seeds Sprouted Radish Seeds • Purslane • Navy Beans Lima Beans • Garden Peas • Oat Germ • Wheat Germ • Corn Germ • Wheat Bran • Almonds Kale • Pinto Beans • Common Beans Walnuts • Pecans

Food Sources of Omega-6 Fatty Acids

Oils containing omega-6 fatty acids, mostly as linoleic acid:

Higher Percentage

Grapeseed Oil • Wheat germ Oil • Corn Oil Walnut Oil • Cottonseed Oil • Sunflower Oil Safflower Oil • Refined Soy Bean Oil • Peanut Oil

Moderate Percentage

Sesame Oil • Sunflower • Rice Bran Oil Canola Oil • Almond Oil

Lower Parcentage

Flax Seed Oil • Avocado Oil • Lard • Hazelnut Oil Olive Oil • Palm Oil • Butter/Ghee • Beef Tallow Macadamia Nut Oil • Coconut Oil Palm Kernel Oil

Omega-3 Enriched Eggs

To increase the omega-3 content found in chicken eggs, hens are fed oils that contain omega-3 fatty acids. Some of the oils used in the chicken's feed include: menhaden, krill, flax seed and algae. The amount and type of omega-3 fatty acids present in an omega-3 enriched egg will vary with the chicken's diet.

REGULATION OF BLOOD SUGAR

Well controlled blood sugar decreases the risk for both cataracts and macular degeneration (AMD), while obesity and type II diabetes increase this risk. To help promote blood sugar regulation, eat foods with *High Dietary Fiber,* a low *Glycemic Index* and a source of *Complete Protein*.

1. High Dietary Fiber

Dietary fiber helps to stabilize blood glucose levels by slowing the absorption of carbohydrates in the gut. Insoluble fiber is nature's "broom" helping to maintain digestive system health. Soluble fiber supports maintenance of healthy blood glucose levels and reduces cholesterol absorption.

Vegetables

Corn • Spirulina • Okra • Carrots
Swiss Chard • Beets • Cauliflower
Parsnips • Zucchini • Eggplant • Celery
French Beans • Lima Beans • Artichoke
Sweet Potato • Broccoli • Brussels Sprouts
Cabbage • Asparagus • Bok Choy • Fennel
Pumpkin • Cooked Kale • Fresh Peas
Butternut Squash • Yellow Squash
Acorn Squash • Spaghetti Squash

Fruits

Passion Fruit • Avocado • Dates
Mullberries • Nectarine • Pineapple
Blueberries • Strawberries • Banana
Blackberries • Boysenberries • Pears
Orange • Cherries • Grapefruit • Papaya
Apples • Cranberries • Starfruit • Mango
Pomegranate • Guava • Raspberries
Plum • Peach • Kiwi

2. Glycemic Index

Glycemic index is a convenient way to measure the relative influence on blood sugar of one food versus a standard food. A food that has a low glycemic index will not raise the blood sugar as quickly as food with a high glycemic index. The portion size of the carbohydrate eaten and its glycemic index are used to calculate the glycemic load. When preparing meals or making food choices, reduce the effect of higher glycemic impact foods by choosing smaller portions or combining with low glycemic index foods and quality protein.

Low (25 or less)

Zucchini • Artichoke • Asparagus
Radish • Broccoli • Eggplant • Onion
Cabbage • Celery • Cucumber • Cherries
Collard Greens • Swiss Chard • Hummus
Tomato • Brussels Sprouts • Soy Beans
Spinach • Romaine Lettuce • Kale
Protein (*Eggs, Meat, Fish, Tofu, Poultry*)
Low or Nonfat Plain Greek Yogurt

Medium-Low (30-55)

Squash • Carrots • Hearts Of Palm
Grapefruit • Dried Apples • Prunes
Cauliflower • Bell Pepper • Green Peas
Mixed Nuts • Whole Meal Spaghetti
Plum • Peach • Tomato Juice • Lentils
Yellow Split Peas • Beans • Whole Milk
Skim Milk • Full-Fat Soy Milk
Dried Apricots • Pear • Apple
Dark Chocolate

Medium (56-69)

Whole Rye Kernel • Whole Kernel Barley
Whole Kernel Buckwheat Bread
Cracked Bulgur • Strawberries
Oranges • Grapes • Pineapple Juice
Brown Rice • Quinoa • Corn on the Cob
Plain Popcorn • Yams • Banana

High (70 and up)

Sweet Potato • White Potato
Watermelon • Rice Cakes
Soda Crackers • Graham Crackers
Agave Nectar • Sucrose (*Table Sugar*)
Cream of Wheat • Bagels
White Rice • Rice Noodles
White Wheat Flour • Honey

3. Complete Protein

Building a meal with complete proteins is important to promote blood sugar regulation. Proteins also help the body to build, maintain and repair itself. Complete proteins are constructed from 22 amino acids. Animal-based foods, such as fish, poultry, meat and eggs contain all 22 amino acids.

Plant-based foods are incomplete protein sources, with the exception of soy and quinoa. However, a meal can be built with a complete source of protein by combining incomplete protein sources. For example:

Grains + Legumes
Brown Rice + Red Beans
Corn + String Beans

Grains + Nuts + Seeds
Whole Grain Bread + Walnuts +
Sunflower Seeds

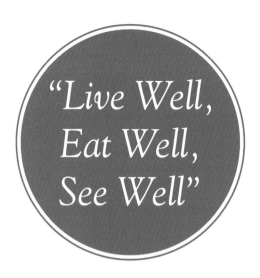

"Live Well, Eat Well, See Well"

Eye health maintenance is supported by factors other than nutrition. There are non-modifiable risk factors for eye disease such as heredity, age, race and gender. There are also modifiable risk factors that increase the possibility of acquiring ocular health issues, such as UV exposure, smoking, lack of exercise and obesity.

UV Exposure

Sunlight can be beneficial to one's health. Sunlight provides much needed vitamin D, as well as giving us a sense of well being. Overexposure to intense UV light can have adverse affects on skin and eyes. Sun damage may lead to premature aging of the skin and skin cancer. Sun damage to eyes increases the risk of developing cataracts, macular degeneration and eye cancer. The carotenoids lutein and zeaxanthin act as a natural sunscreen. Eating foods rich in these nutrients may help to protect the macula from UV damage. In high intensity midday sunlight, it is best to wear sunglasses that provide UV and blue light protection labeled: UV 400.

Smoking Cessation

Cigarette smoking not only increases the risk for developing lung cancer and heart disease, it also increases the likelihood of developing macular degeneration (AMD). Continued smoking with macular degeneration increases the risk of progression. Please note that current and former smokers should not take vitamin supplements with beta-carotene, as it increases the risk of developing lung cancer.

Smoking is also a risk factor for developing cataracts. Also, lower vitamin C levels found in ocular tissues of smokers may contribute to oxidative stress leading to cataract formation

Exercise

Studies have shown that regular exercise may reduce the risk for developing cataracts and macular degeneration. Exercising regularly at least three times each week may help to slow down the progression of macular degeneration. Physical activity supports general health and well being, reducing the risk of cardiovascular disease and stroke. Please check with your physician before starting an exercise regimen.

Weight Management

Obesity is linked to an increased risk of developing several vision threatening diseases: diabetic retinopathy, cataracts, glaucoma and macular degeneration. Exercise and eating a low glycemic impact diet, rich in antioxidants and omega-3 fatty acids, will help a person to achieve a healthful weight.

Lifetime of Wellness

The choices we make can have a positive or negative effect on our bodies over a lifetime. Nutrition, exercise, attitude and alcohol/drug use, added up over time can influence how we age. Taking care of ourselves through the years, both nutritionally and physically, can lead to a higher quality of life. Some health ailments associated with age may be lessened or delayed. Could nutrition and lifestyle improve vision and balance, decrease falls and fractures as we age? Let's all strive for healthy golden years!

COMMON DISEASES OF THE EYE

Two of the most common eye diseases that effect Americans are Age-related Macular Degeneration (AMD) and cataracts. Nutrition has been shown to have an affect on both of these eye health problems.

Macular Degeneration

Age-related Macular Degeneration (AMD) is an eye disease which slowly and painlessly reduces central vision. In the back of the eye, there is a light sensitive tissue known as the retina. The retina is made up of light-sensitive cells known as rods and cones. The retina receives light energy and converts it into bioelectrical signals which are then sent to the brain for interpretation as vision. The central portion of the retina is called the macula. The macula consists mainly of cone cells. Cone cells are responsible for color vision, daytime vision, and our ability to see fine detail.

As we age, the cells in the macula can deteriorate prematurely resulting in AMD. AMD can progress slowly ("dry AMD") or quickly ("wet AMD"). Macular degeneration can reduce or eliminate a person's ability to see faces, read without special vision aids or drive. People with AMD normally retain their peripheral vision, allowing them to continue to participate in other activities of daily life.

Macular degeneration affects more than 10 million people in the United States and is the leading cause of vision loss and blindness among Americans aged 65 and older. The incidence of AMD increases with each decade of life over the age of 50. AMD has both genetic and environmental causes. The lifetime risk of developing late stage AMD is 50% for those who have a relative with AMD, and drops to 12% for those without a relative with AMD. While heredity is not normally modifiable, many environmental factors that increase the risk of developing AMD are modifiable.

Steps that can be taken to help reduce the risk for developing AMD include:

- Stop smoking
- Wear sunglasses providing UV and blue light protection
- Healthy weight maintenance
- Regular Exercise
- Proper diet and nutrition

Recent research has shown that a diet rich in the carotenoids lutein and zeaxanthin, the omega-3 fatty acids DHA/EPA, vitamins A, C and E, the mineral zinc, and dietary fiber may help to reduce the risk of progression of AMD.

Cataracts

A cataract is a clouding of the lens inside the eye which can lead to decreased vision. The cloudy lens can be described as looking through a dirty window, causing difficulty with glare sensitivity and seeing details of an object. Although there are many different types of cataracts, age-related cataracts are by far the most common form. Cataracts affect nearly 22 million Americans age 40 and older. By age 80, more than half of all Americans have or have had cataracts.

Although heredity plays a role in age-related cataract formation, certain environmental factors have been shown to increase the risk for the development of cataracts. Excessive exposure to bright sunlight over time, cigarette smoking and certain drugs, such as corticosteroids, can induce cataract formation in some people.

Recent research has shown a potentially protective effect of diets rich in the carotenoids lutein and zeaxanthin on the risk of developing cataracts. Omega-3 fatty acids may also support lens health.

Human Eye Anatomy

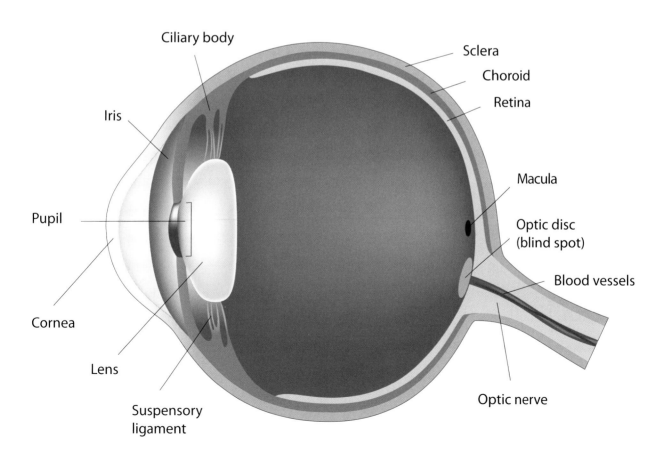

Alila Medical Media/Shutterstock

COOKING PRACTICES

Select Quality Cookware

When sautéing, select a pan with a ceramic, non-stick surface. The pan should have a well-fitting lid. The ceramic surface is food safe to 550°F and minimizes the amount of oil needed. Non-reactive, heavy gauge, stainless steel or enameled (*pictured*) cookware are both ideally suited for extended cooking times. To help recapture and retain nutrients while cooking, cover the pan as often as possible.

How to Heat Your Skillet

Patiently bring a skillet or Dutch oven up to the lowest heat required for the recipe. Add the oil followed by the other ingredients immediately. This will minimize heat damage to the oil being used. Many chefs advocate bringing the temperature of the pan to "screaming hot". This is not a healthful practice. A sauté pan preheated to medium or medium-high will create an environment that produces delicious foods without damaging the nutrients.

Cooking Time & Temperature

Higher heat and extended amounts of time used to cook food degrade heat sensitive nutrients such as vitamins A, C, E and the omega-3 fatty acids. Minerals will not be lost during extended cooking. The amount of water used for cooking can impact the preservation and concentration of antioxidants. Boiling carrots in water versus steaming or lightly sautéing will reduce the amount of beta-carotene retained in the carrots.

Why Wash Your Produce?

Produce, both organically and conventionally grown, needs to be washed before consumption. All produce can have pathogens and dirt which should be removed. Conventionally grown produce has the added burden of pesticide residues. Pesticide residues tend to concentrate in the peel. Vitamins and micronutrients tend to concentrate in the peel as well. Peeling conventionally grown produce diminishes exposure to the residues. With certain produce, such as celery, it is not possible to wash or peel away these residues. Consume organically grown produce whenever possible.

Maximizing Bioavailability & Nutritional Content

The fat soluble vitamins are more efficiently absorbed by our bodies when consumed with a fat. The vitamin A family as well as the vitamins D, E and K are all fat soluble. Important to eye health are lutein, zeaxanthin, lycopene and beta-carotene; all part of the fat soluble vitamin A family.

To maximize the absorption of the carotenoids found in tomatoes, consider consuming with avocados using the recipes for Salsa Fresca (page 189) and Guacamole (page 189). Kale and olive oil are combined in the Turmeric Pearl Onions & Kale (page 160).

Steaming, sautéing or pureeing vegetables will break down the plant cell walls, increasing the body's access to these nutrients. For the recipes in this cookbook, many of the fruits and vegetables are not peeled, so as to preserve as many of the nutrients and dietary fiber as possible.

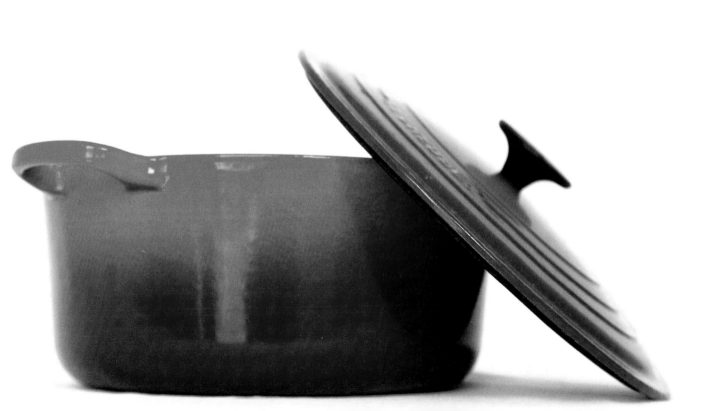

PANTRY ESSENTIALS

PRODUCE

Orange Bell Pepper • Kale • Spinach • Onion
Garlic • Shallots • Broccoli • Green Beans
Asparagus • Cabbage • Romaine Lettuce
Mustard Greens • Brussels Sprouts • Beets
Cauliflower • Artichokes • Cucumber • Ginger
Mushrooms (*Crimini, Shiitake, Porcini,
Portabello*) • Zucchini • Carrot • Yellow Squash
Celery • Hot Peppers • Corn on the Cob
Sweet Potatoes • Strawberries • Blueberries
Raspberries • Blackberries • Honeydew Melon
Kiwi • Mangoes • Nectarines • Peach • Apple
Apricot • Passionfruit

PROTEIN

Salmon (*Wild, Canned, Smoked, Sockeye, King,
Coho*) • Rainbow Trout • Tilapia • Striped Bass
Mussels • Oysters • Crab • Scallops
Grass-Fed Beef • Free Range Poultry
Lamb Venison • Bison, Calf & Turkey Liver
Non-GMO Tofu (*Firm, Extra-Firm, Silken-Firm*)

ORGANIC DAIRY & EGGS

Grass-Fed Cheese • Plain Greek Yogurt
Omega-3 Eggs • Nondairy Soymilk
Nondairy Soy Products

CANNED GOODS

Tomatoes, Whole Or Diced • Tomato Paste
Chickpeas • Black Beans • Kidney Beans
Cannellini Beans • Artichokes • Pumpkin Puree
Coconut Milk (Light or Regular)
Wild Alaskan Salmon • Sardines • Anchovies

NUTS & SEEDS

Walnuts • Almonds • Flax Seeds • Pepita Seeds
Sunflower Seeds • Sesame Seeds

ORGANIC OILS

First Cold-Press Extra Virgin Olive Oil
Coconut Oil • Expeller-Pressed Canola Oil
Dark Sesame Oil

CONDIMENTS

Asian Dark Vinegar • Red Wine Vinegar

Apple Cider Vinegar • Organic Ketchup

Balsamic Vinegar • Rice Vinegar • Hot Sauce

Whole Grain Mustard • Soy Sauce or Tamari

Raw Honey • Maple Syrup • Agave Nectar

STAPLES

Black Beans • Kidney Beans • Chickpeas

Quinoa • Farro • Wild Rice • Brown Rice

Buckwheat Noodles • Whole Grain Pasta • Lentils

Sun Dried Tomatoes • Dehydrated Mushrooms

Polenta Style Cornmeal

BAKING

Natural Cocoa Powder • Cacao Nibs

Dark Chocolate (70% or Higher)

Dried Fruit (Blueberries, Cranberries,

Tart Cherries, Apricots, Goldenberries,

Raisins and Dates)

HERBS & SPICES

Iodized Sea Salt • Black Peppercorns

Red Pepper Flakes • Paprika (*Smoked or Sweet*)

Garlic Powder • Onion Powder • Fennel

Cilantro • Parsley • Oregano • Rosemary

Thyme • Sage • Italian Herb Blend

Bouquet Garni • Turmeric • Garam Masala

Coriander • Cumin • Ginger • Cinnamon

Star Anise • Cloves • Nutmeg • Cardamom

Chili Powder • Achiote Seeds

TEA

Green Tea Bags • Matcha Powder

Hibiscus or Rose Hip Tea

FROZEN

Blueberries • Raspberries • Strawberries

Green Beans • Corn • Edamame

Salmon (*King, Sockeye or Coho*)

Lemon or Lime Juice

"Eye Spice" Cubes (page 205)

Coconut Milk Cubes (page 205)

Homemade Stock In User-Friendly

Portion Size (page 93)

HARDWARE

High-Speed Blender • Food Processor

Immersion Blender

Covered Ceramic Nonstick Sauté Pan

Heavy Dutch Oven, 5-7 Quart Size

Large Lidded Stock Pot

Covered Sauce Pots (*Small and Large*)

Mixing Bowls • Measuring Cups and Spoons

Cheese Grater • Extra Wide Vegetable Peeler

Salad Spinner • Coffee or Spice Grinder

Mortar And Pestle • Tongs • Whisks

Spatula • Pancake Turner • Strainer • Colander

Fine Mesh Strainer • Non-Stick Baking Sheet

Glass Bakewear (10"×15"×2") and (9"×7"×2.5")

Fat Separator • Hand or Stand Mixer

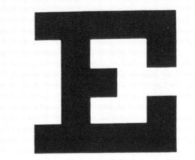

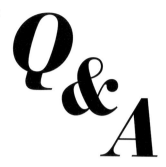 **with the Author, Sandra Young, OD**

Dr. Young, why did you decide to write a cookbook for eye health?

There has been a recent explosion of research into eye health and nutrition and the results have been encouraging. I wanted to share this science with others in a practical way, through diet and tasty recipes aimed at enhancing eye health. There is an ever increasing number of Americans who are visually impaired by cataracts, type 2 diabetes and macular degeneration. While there are genetic components, diet and lifestyle can alter the risk of visual impairment. This cookbook fills a need for good tasting, user-friendly recipes. My readers will be able to use these recipes every day of the week, all year long. Proper nutrition gives the eyes, as well as the body, the "tools" to have the best opportunity to maintain a great quality of life through our important sense of vision.

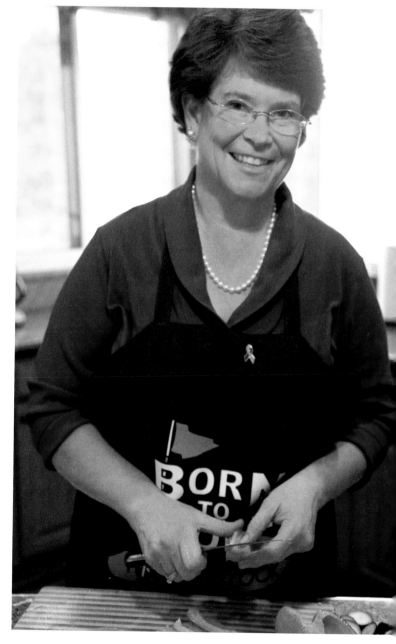

How did you create these tasty recipes?

I went backwards! First, I looked at the science of nutrition and eye health. Then I began to research what a balanced eye diet should include. I knew that the cornerstone of these recipes had to be anti-inflammatory and "eye nutrient" dense. Also, the recipes should promote level blood sugar values through fiber and quality protein, emphasizing omega-3 fatty acids. I compiled lists of foods based upon their specific nutrient densities and health benefits. The recipes were created from these lists. I include the lists to allow each person to individualize their meals while eating the most nutritious foods for their eye health.

Macular degeneration (Age-related Macular Degeneration or AMD) and cataracts are two of the leading causes of visual impairment in Americans. Will diet and lifestyle really help their vision?

Yes. Recent studies have shown that proper diet and exercise have the power to alter the course of macular degeneration in many people. While there are hereditary components, nutrition and lifestyle play a role in decreasing the risk of visual impairment with age. Research has shown that the carotenoids lutein and zeaxanthin, and the antioxidants vitamins C and E, in combination with beta-carotene, zinc and the omega-3 fatty acids play a supporting role in maintaining good ocular health. Acquiring these nutrients in a whole food form creates a beneficial nutritional synergy for our eyes beyond what supplements alone can provide. Lifestyle can promote healthier eyes and better vision. A healthful "eye diet" promotes level blood sugar and a healthy weight. This should be complimented with

regular physical activity. Smoking is a risk factor for developing macular degeneration (AMD). Wearing quality UV400 protective sunglasses helps to lessen the stress ultraviolet light places on the macula. There are indications that these measures are also likely to delay or reduce the risk of cataract formation in many individuals.

Are there other health benefits associated with eating these foods beyond ocular health?

A diet that is good for the eyes is also good for several organ systems as well as overall health. The retina, a neurological layer inside the eye comprised of light receptors, is an "outcropping" of the brain. The brain and the retina both benefit from eating fish high in omega-3 fatty acids regularly. A diet high in omega-3's may slow the progression of cognitive decline in Alzheimer's patients and even improve mental skills. Omega-3's and the antioxidants in an "eye diet" decrease the risk for certain cancers and chronic inflammatory diseases. The lower glycemic impact foods and complex carbohydrates decrease the risk of developing type 2 diabetes. These same nutritional principles are considered beneficial for cardiovascular health.

Macular degeneration runs in my family. Will providing my children with a good "eye diet" help their eyes?

A diet containing the carotenoids, lutein and zeaxanthin, as well as omega-3's are important for healthy neurological development of the eyes and the brain. The need for these nutrients starts early as they are components of breast milk. Years of "empty" nutrition can have negative long term consequences on vision and general health. Since macular degeneration runs in families, it is especially important for children and young adults to include these nutrient dense foods as part of their regular diet. When an older family member has been diagnosed with macular degeneration, the value of these recommendations are likely to be even more critical.

Should I eat "eye nutritious" foods before and after eye surgery?

It is important to keep your eyes and your body as healthy as possible so they can recover more easily from surgery, stress or toxins. Ocular tissues armed with the right nutrients in place have a better chance for a good surgical outcome. However, certain foods, like kale, parsley and garlic may increase the risk of certain surgical complications. It is imperative to discuss with your eye surgeon all medications, supplements and certain foods that are ingested before and after surgery. Individuals with special medical or dietary needs should always discuss these with their physician.

Dr. Young, I see your recipes include many herbs and spices -- why?

Besides making food taste great, herbs and spices are power-packed with micronutrients and antioxidants. They have eye health benefits -- paprika contains vitamin A, lutein and zeaxanthin, rosemary has been shown to support retinal health, parsley is an excellent source of vitamins A, C and K, as well as beta-carotene, lutein and zeaxanthin. Turmeric and ginger are delicious anti-inflammatories. Cinnamon helps to promote balanced blood sugar.

What is your cooking and culinary background?

My family has a great culinary tradition, blending the Mediterrenean flavors of Southern Italy and France with the cuisines of New Orleans. I love using the traditional ingredients from these areas. You'll find that many of the ingredients and spices in the recipes created for *Visionary Kitchen* have come from these regions. I have been a home chef, cooking for my family and friends for over 45 years. Many decades ago, I had to decide between going to optometry school and culinary school. This cookbook combines my passion for cooking with my profession of eye care.

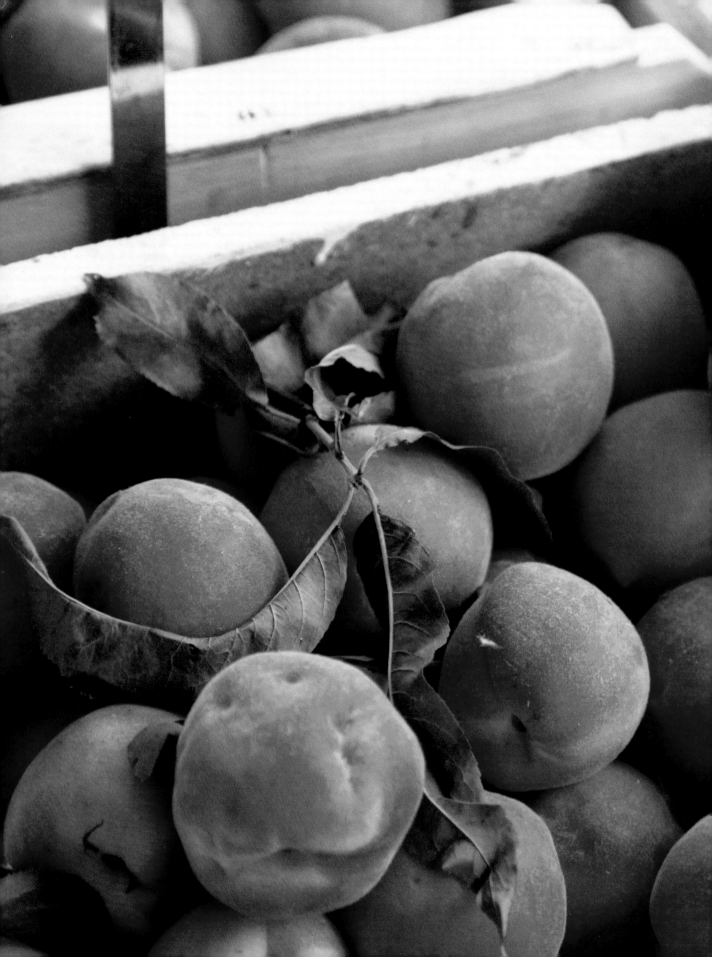

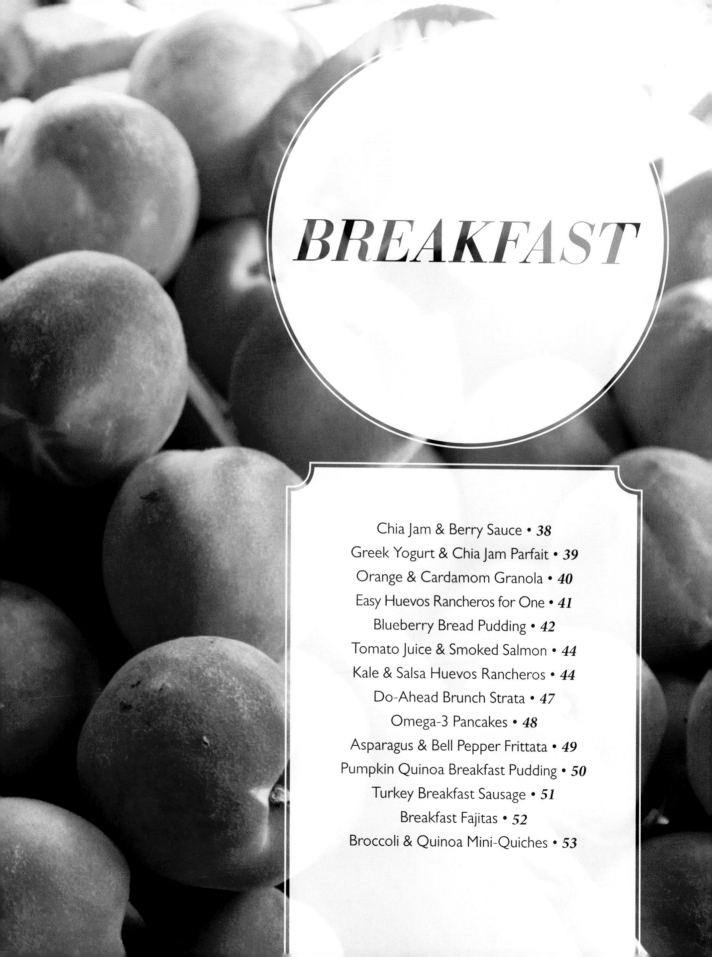

BREAKFAST

Chia Jam & Berry Sauce

A superfood packed jam with no added sugar, no cooking, and plenty of flavor. Chia seeds absorb more than 10 times their weight in liquid at room temperature, giving this jam a wonderfully spreadable consistency.

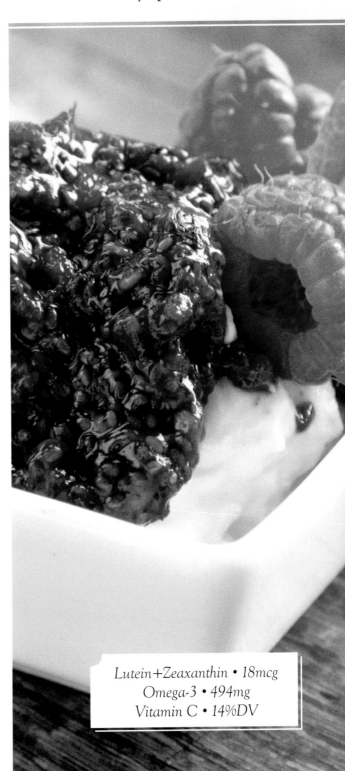

chia jam

- 2 cups organic berries, fresh or frozen, thawed
- 2½ Tbsp chia seeds
- 2 tsp açaí powder or lemon juice
- 1-2 tsp raw honey, optional

chia berry sauce

- 2 cups organic berries, fresh or frozen, thawed
- 1½ Tbsp chia seeds
- 2 tsp açaí powder or lemon juice
- 1-2 tsp raw honey, optional

1. For either chia jam or sauce, use an immersion blender to puree the berries to a smooth consistency. The berry puree should measure 1 to 1¼ cups.

2. Stir in the chia seeds and allow to sit for 30 minutes.

3. Stir in the açaí powder or lemon juice and taste. If the berries are too tart, consider adding a little honey.

MAKES 1½ CUPS • SERVES 12

Consider using the berry chia jam on Greek yogurt, in a smoothie, or on a slice of whole grain toast "buttered" with 1 tsp coconut oil.

Lutein+Zeaxanthin • 18mcg
Omega-3 • 494mg
Vitamin C • 14%DV

Omega-3 • 2,848mg
Folate • 21%DV
Zinc • 32%DV

Greek Yogurt & Chia Jam Parfait

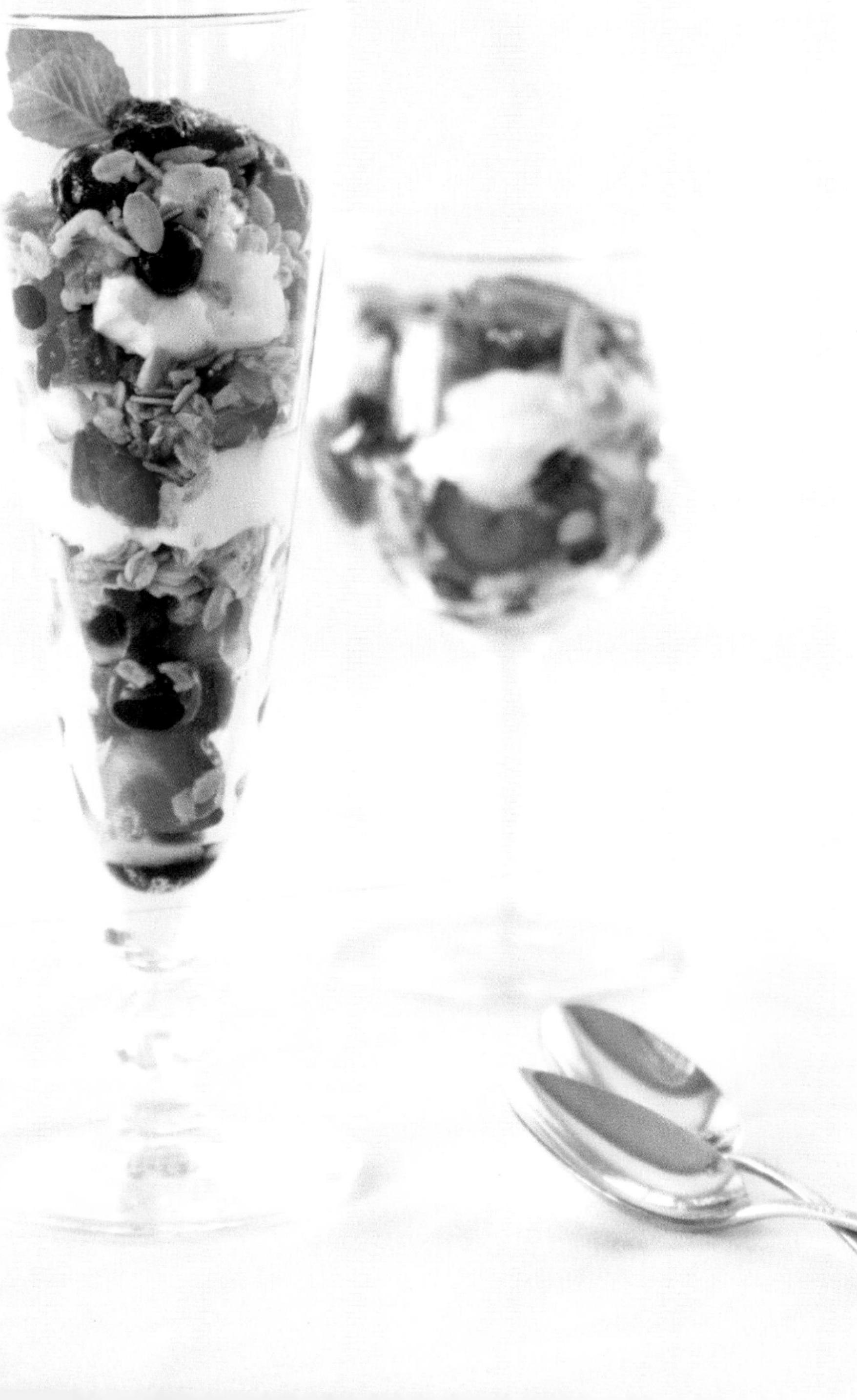

¾ cup plain Greek yogurt
¼ cup Chia Jam (page 38)
½ cup fresh berries
⅓ cup Orange & Cardamom Granola (page 40)

Sprig of fresh mint, for garnish

1. To the bottom of a parfait glass, add half of the yogurt, Chia Jam, fresh berries and granola.

2. Repeat, finishing with a layer of fresh berries. Garnish with mint if desired.

SERVES 1

Raspberries have fiber and antioxidants. Nonfat Greek yogurt contains lots of protein to maintain steady blood glucose.

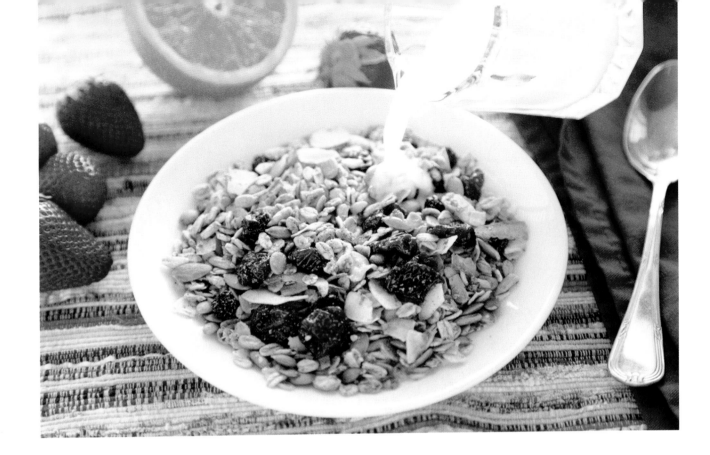

Orange & Cardamom Granola

4 cups old-fashioned rolled oats

1½ cups unsweetened coconut flakes

½ cup pepita seeds

1½ cups walnuts, chopped

½ cup sunflower seeds

2 tsp cinnamon

½ tsp ground cardamom

1 tsp orange zest

⅓ cup orange juice

½ cup maple syrup

2 tsp vanilla extract

½ tsp sea salt

3 Tbsp organic coconut oil, melted

½ cup flax seed, ground

1½ cups dried fruit, roughly chopped (blueberries, cherries, apricots, goldenberries, goji berries or cranberries)

1. Preheat oven to 300°F. Combine the first 13 ingredients in an extra large mixing bowl.

2. Pour melted coconut oil over the oat mixture. Pour over the oat mixture. Stir well to coat evenly.

3. Pour oat mixture onto a baking sheet. Toast in the oven, stirring every 10 minutes until golden and fragrant, 50-60 minutes. Stir in ground flax seed the last 10 minutes.

4. Remove from oven, and while still warm, stir in the dried fruit. After completely cooled, store in an air-tight container.

MAKES 9½ CUPS • 22 SERVINGS

Lutein+Zeaxanthin • 18mcg
Folate • 8%DV
Zinc • 14%DV

Easy Huevos Rancheros for One

with egg

⅓ cup frozen spinach,
   thawed and drained
¼ tsp turmeric
Sea salt & black pepper,
   to taste
⅓ cup Salsa Fresca (page 189)
I omega-3 egg
¼ cup tomato, diced
I Tbsp organic
   cheddar cheese, optional

Lutein+Zeaxanthin • 9,138mcg
Omega-3 • 464mg
Lycopene • 2,229mcg

1. Preheat oven to 350°F. In small bowl, mix spinach, turmeric and salsa. Add the spinach mixture to a 1-pint sized oven safe dish, forming a well in the center.

2. Crack the egg into the well, cover with foil and bake for 15 minutes.

3. Remove the foil and continue to bake another 5-10 minutes until the egg is set.

4. Garnish with diced tomatoes and cheese.

with tofu

½ cup extra-firm tofu,
   drained
¼ tsp turmeric
Pinch onion powder
Sea salt & black pepper,
   to taste
⅓ cup frozen spinach,
   thawed and drained
⅓ cup Salsa Fresca (page 189)
I tsp extra virgin olive oil
¼ cup tomato, diced

Lycopene • 2,119mcg
Lutein+Zeaxanthin • 8,972mcg
Vitamin E • 16%DV

1. Preheat oven to 350°F. Crumble the tofu into a small dish. Add turmeric, onion powder, salt and pepper to the tofu. Stir well.

2. In another bowl, mix spinach, salsa and olive oil.

3. Add the spinach mixture to a 1-pint sized oven safe dish, forming a well in the center. Spoon the tofu mixture into the well. Bake until heated through, about 10 minutes. Garnish with diced tomatoes.

4. Alternately, microwave 1-2 minutes until hot.

Blueberry Bread Pudding

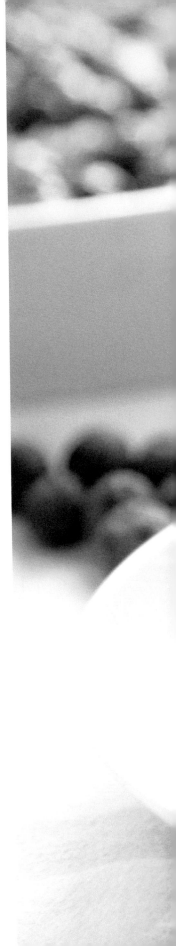

4 large omega-3 eggs
¼ cup maple syrup
¾ cup organic milk of choice
1 tsp cinnamon
Pinch cardamom
½ tsp vanilla extract
½ cup plain Greek yogurt
4 slices hearty whole grain bread

2 cups blueberries, fresh or frozen
1 tsp coconut sugar

⅓ cup walnuts, for garnish
1 ½ cups plain Greek yogurt, for garnish

8"×8" baking dish

1. In a mixing bowl, beat eggs, maple syrup, milk, cinnamon, cardamom, vanilla extract and Greek yogurt.

2. Tear bread into chunks and stir gently into egg mixture. Pour into a lightly greased 8"×8" baking dish and allow to sit at least 30 minutes or overnight in the refrigerator.

3. Preheat oven to 350°F. Just before baking, top bread mixture with the blueberries, then sprinkle with coconut sugar for an added crunch. Bake for 40 minutes or until the center has risen and a tester comes out clean.

4. To serve, portion an amount onto a plate and top with lightly roasted walnuts (page 213) and ¼ cup Greek yogurt.

SERVES 6

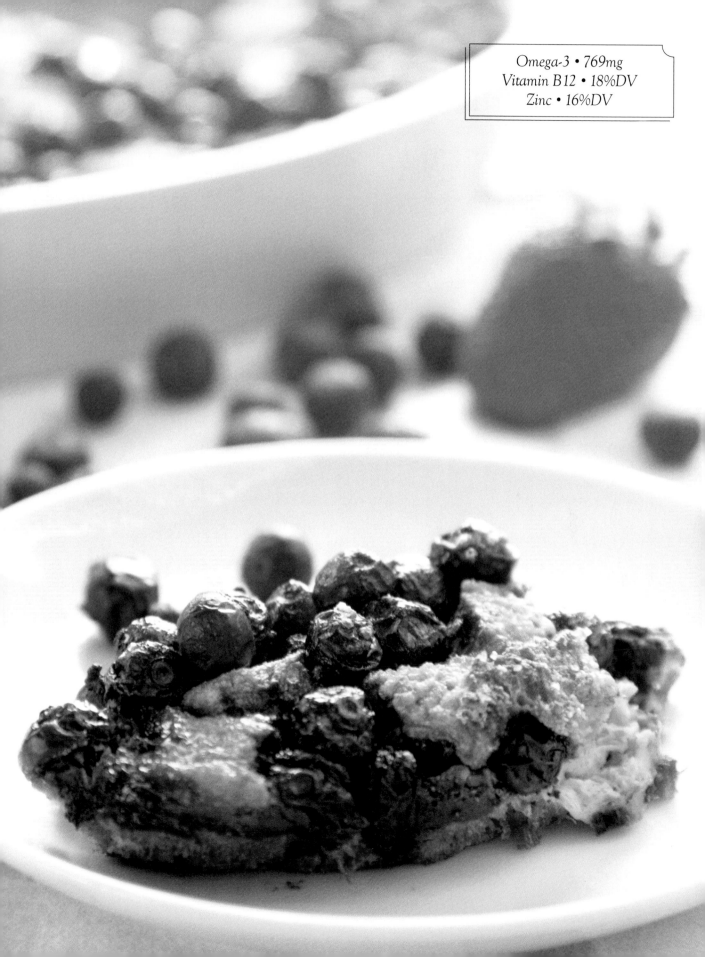

Omega-3 • 769mg
Vitamin B12 • 18%DV
Zinc • 16%DV

Tomato Juice & Smoked Salmon

3 cups vine-ripened
  tomatoes, quartered
¼ cup celery with leaves,
  coarsely chopped
¼ cup orange bell pepper,
  coarsely chopped
⅓ cup broccoli, coarsely
  chopped
½ cup cucumber, peeled and
  coarsely chopped
2 Tbsp onion, diced
¼ garlic clove
1 sprig parsley
¼ tsp paprika,
  sweet or smoked

1 tsp Worcestershire sauce
2-3 shakes hot sauce
⅛ tsp black pepper
Sea salt, to taste
½ tsp oregano,
  fresh or dried
¼ cup filtered water

Juice of 1 lime

serve with

8 oz smoked salmon
8 high fiber whole-grain
  crackers, gluten free if
  desired

1. Place all ingredients into a high-speed blender and puree until smooth.

2. Pour tomato juice into glasses and serve with high-fiber crackers and smoked salmon.

MAKES 3½ CUPS • SERVES 4

Lycopene • 3,474mcg
Omega-3 • 1,237mg
Vitamin C • 69%DV

Kale & Salsa Huevos Rancheros

recipe continued on next page ›››

1 onion, diced
1 garlic clove, minced
1 Tbsp extra virgin
  olive oil

1 lb kale, coarsely
  chopped

¼ cup light
  coconut milk
1 tsp turmeric
4 oz can diced green
  chilies
2 cups Salsa Fresca
  (page 189)

½ tsp sea salt
½ tsp black pepper

6 omega-3 eggs
½ cup organic cheddar
  cheese, grated

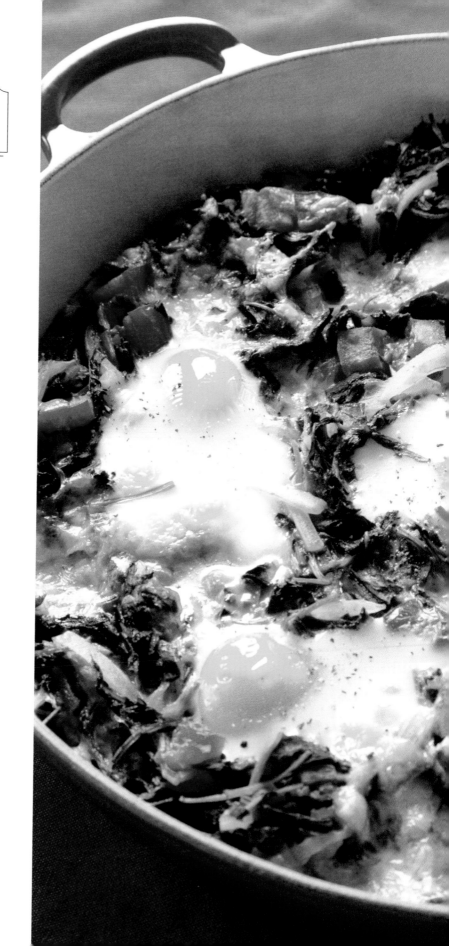

Lutein+Zeaxanthin • 29,878mcg
Omega-3 • 416mg
Vitamin C • 177%DV

1. Preheat oven to 350°F. Preheat a 12" oven-safe sauté pan to medium. Sauté onion and garlic in olive oil for 3-5 minutes or until the onion softens and takes on a little color.

2. Add kale, coconut milk, turmeric, green chilies, salsa, salt and pepper; stir to combine. Continue to sauté until mixture is heated through and kale has wilted. Remove from heat.

3. Using 2 forks, create 6 small wells in the cooked kale. Crack one egg into each well. Cover the sauté pan with a lid or aluminum foil.

4. Bake for 30 minutes. Uncover and continue to bake until the egg yolks are set and cooked to desired doneness.

5. Remove from oven and sprinkle with cheese. Partially cover for 1-2 minutes to allow cheese to melt. Serve immediately.

SERVES 6

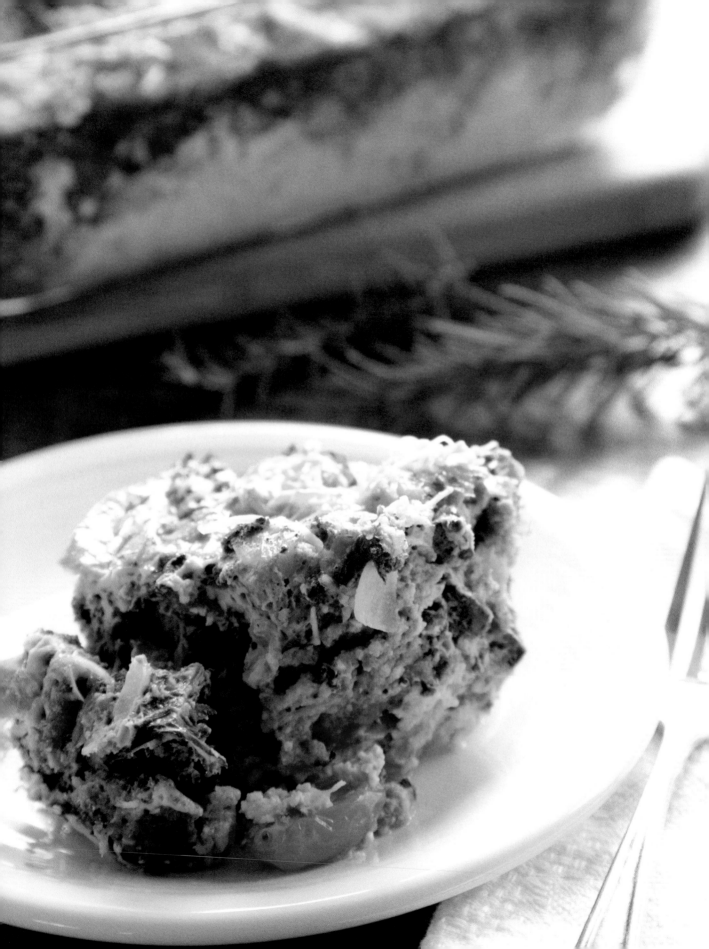

Do-Ahead Brunch Strata

1 ¼ cups onion, small dice
1 garlic clove, minced
1 Tbsp extra virgin olive oil

2 cups mushrooms, sliced
3 cups kale, finely chopped
¾ cup roasted bell pepper
(page 179), cut into strips

8 omega-3 eggs
2 cups organic milk
of choice
½ tsp sea salt
¼ tsp black pepper
½ tsp turmeric
4 cups hearty whole grain
bread, cubed (day old is
best)

½ cup cherry tomatoes,
halved
½ cup parmesan or
romano cheese, grated

9"×12" baking dish, greased

1. Preheat a large sauté pan over medium, add olive oil quickly followed by the garlic and onion. Sauté until softened, 3-5 minutes. Add mushrooms, kale and bell pepper; sauté an additional 3-5 minutes. Remove from the heat and allow to cool.

2. In a mixing bowl, mix eggs, milk, salt, pepper and turmeric. Add kale mixture to the egg and milk mixture. Add bread cubes and gently stir to combine.

3. Pour into prepared baking dish. Allow to sit 1 hour or overnight in the refrigerator.

4. Preheat oven to 350°F. Evenly place tomatoes on top, sprinkle with cheese. Bake uncovered for 45-55 minutes until puffed and golden. A tester should come out clean.

SERVES 12

Variation: Stir in ½ recipe cooked Turkey Breakfast Sausage (page 51).

Lutein+Zeaxanthin • 6,762mcg
Omega-3 • 207mg
Zinc • 9%DV

Omega-3 Pancakes

½ cup old fashioned oats
¼ cup walnuts
½ cup whole wheat flour
¼ tsp sea salt
2 Tbsp ground flax seed
2 Tbsp wheat germ
½ tsp cinnamon
1 tsp baking powder
¼ tsp baking soda

2 omega-3 eggs
1½ Tbsp maple syrup
⅔ cup organic milk of choice
1½ Tbsp organic cold-pressed canola oil
¼ cup plain Greek yogurt

1 cup organic Greek yogurt
½ cup Chia Jam (page 38)

1. Grind oatmeal and walnuts in food processor to make a rustic flour. Place walnut-oat flour in a large mixing bowl.

2. Add wheat flour, salt, flax, wheat germ, cinnamon, baking powder and baking soda.

3. In another bowl, combine eggs, maple syrup, milk, canola oil and yogurt; whisk to combine.

4. Add the liquid ingredients to the dry ingredients. Gently stir to combine. Let batter stand for 10 minutes before using.

5. Heat a lightly greased griddle to 300°F. Ladle ¼ cup of the batter onto the griddle, flipping after 2-3 minutes when bubbles begin to form on top, until golden browned.

6. Serve with Greek yogurt, Chia Jam and fresh fruit.

MAKES 12-14 PANCAKES • SERVES 4

Omega-3 • 2,500mg
Vitamin B12 • 16%DV
Zinc • 22%DV

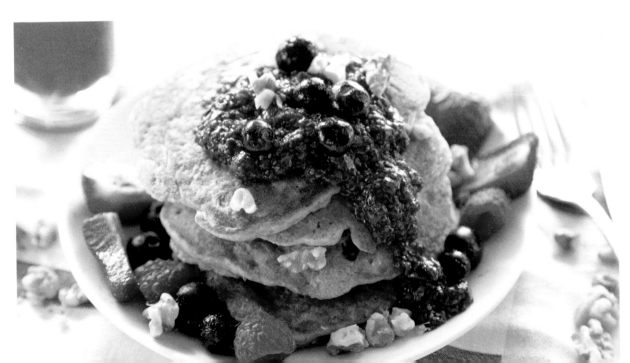

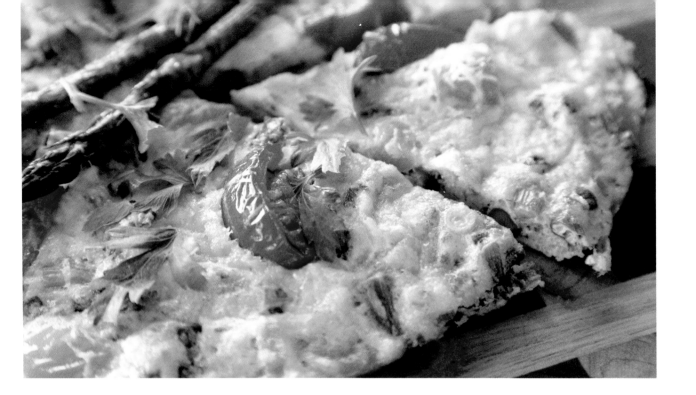

Asparagus & Bell Pepper Frittata

7 omega-3 eggs
2 Tbsp water
3 Tbsp fresh parsley, minced
3 scallions, finely minced
¼ tsp sea salt
¼ tsp black pepper

1 orange bell pepper, diced
7 spears asparagus, diced
1 garlic clove, finely minced
1 Tbsp extra virgin olive oil

1 Roma tomato, diced
½ cup freshly grated Romano or Parmesan cheese

10-inch nonstick oven-safe skillet

1. In a mixing bowl, whisk together eggs, water, parsley, scallions, salt and pepper. Set aside. Preheat oven to 375°F.

2. Preheat an oven safe sauté pan to medium. Sauté pepper, asparagus, and garlic in olive oil until softened, 2-3 minutes.

3. Reduce the heat to medium-low and pour egg mixture into the pan. Gently stir eggs occasionally, tilting the pan to allow the uncooked eggs to run toward the edges until the eggs begin to set.

4. Decorate with tomatoes and sprinkle with cheese. Bake until puffed and golden, approximately 10-12 minutes.

5. Slice frittata into 6 wedges. Garnish with additional parsley, if desired.

SERVES 6

Lutein+Zeaxanthin • 513mcg
Omega-3 • 305mg
Vitamin B12 • 16%DV

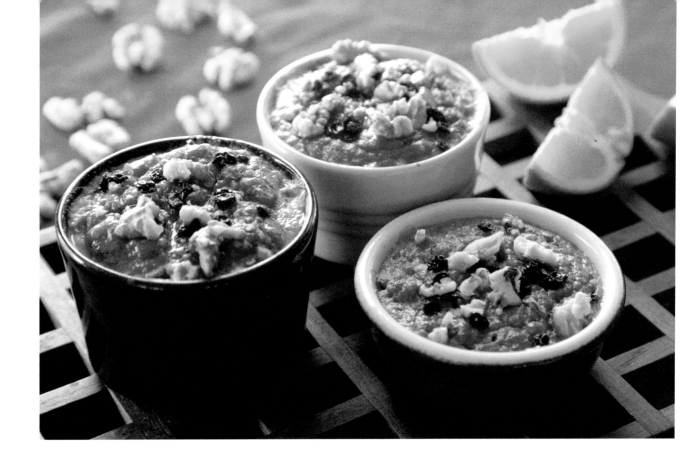

Pumpkin Quinoa Breakfast Pudding

1 cup pumpkin puree
4 omega-3 eggs
1 cup cooked quinoa,
    cooled (page 166)
2 Tbsp light coconut milk
¼ cup maple syrup
¼ cup orange juice
¼ tsp orange zest
2 tsp cinnamon
¼ tsp nutmeg

1 tsp powdered ginger
½ tsp white pepper
¼ tsp sea salt
⅓ cup currants
¼ cup walnuts,
    roughly chopped

6 lightly oiled
    custard cups

Beta-Carotene • 2,846mcg
Omega-3 • 589mg
Zinc • 11%DV

1. Preheat oven to 350°F. Mix all ingredients together in a large mixing bowl.

2. Pour into single-serving greased baking cups. It is best to bake and serve in mini ramekins.

3. Bake until tester comes out clean, about 20 minutes, depending upon the size of the ramekin chosen.

SERVES 6

For an additional omega-3 punch, stir in 2 Tbsp ground flax seed.

Turkey Breakfast Sausage

- 1 lb lean ground turkey, dark meat or 93% lean white meat
- 4 crimini or shiitake mushrooms, chopped into pea-sized pieces
- ¼ cup Italian flat leaf parsley, minced
- 1 garlic clove, finely minced
- 1 tsp turmeric
- 1 tsp dried bouquet garni

- 1 tsp fennel seeds
- 1 tsp sweet paprika
- ¼-½ tsp cayenne pepper, optional
- ¼ tsp black pepper
- ¾ tsp sea salt
- 2 tsp balsamic vinegar

- 1 tsp extra virgin olive oil
- 2 tsp water

1. Place all ingredients in a mixing bowl, except for olive oil and water.

2. Using your hands, completely mix together and shape into 10 small flat patties. Wash your hands thoroughly.

3. Preheat a skillet to medium. Drizzle the pan with olive oil quickly followed by the turkey patties. Brown for approximately 5-6 minutes. Turn over and brown for an additional 2-3 minutes.

4. Add water, and partially cover skillet with a lid. Cook for 3 minutes. Remove the lid, cook 1 more minute. Serve.

MAKES 10 PATTIES

Beta-Carotene • 150mcg
Vitamin B6 • 14%DV
Zinc • 5%DV

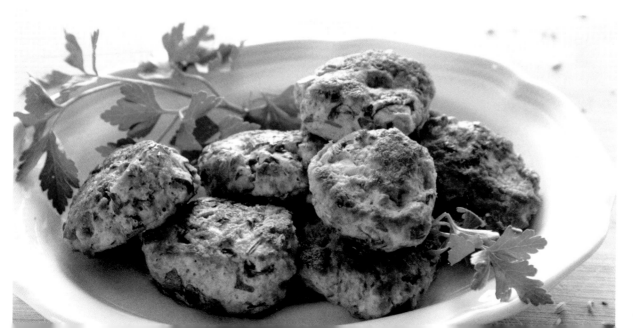

Breakfast Fajitas

2 Tbsp extra virgin olive oil, divided

1 small sweet potato, ¼" dice

15 oz can black beans, drained and rinsed

1 tsp smoked paprika

1 garlic clove, minced

1 medium onion, diced

2 orange bell peppers, cut into strips

½ jalapeño, ribs and seeds removed, small dice

¼ cup cilantro, chopped

1 lb extra firm tofu, drained

¾ tsp turmeric

¼ tsp ground cumin

⅛ tsp onion powder

½ tsp sea salt

¼ tsp black pepper

1 cup diced tomatoes or Salsa Fresca (page 189)

¾ cup plain Greek yogurt

½ avocado, diced

6 large whole-grain tortillas, wrapped in foil

1. Place tortillas in a 250°F oven to warm.

2. Preheat a large sauté pan to medium. Add 1 Tbsp olive oil and the sweet potato. Sauté about 10 minutes until the sweet potato softens and begins to brown. Add black beans and paprika. Stir to combine. Sauté until heated through. Set aside and keep warm.

3. Add the remaining 1 Tbsp of oil to the pan followed by the garlic, onion, bell pepper and jalapeño. Sauté until the vegetables are crisp tender, 8-10 minutes. Remove from the heat and stir in the cilantro.

4. Crumble the tofu into a mixing bowl. Add turmeric, cumin, onion powder, salt and pepper. Stir well to combine. In a non-stick skillet over medium-low, heat the mixture thoroughly. Alternately, microwave to heat.

5. Serve warmed tortillas with the sweet potato-bean mixture, sauted vegetables and tofu. Serve with tomatoes or salsa, Greek yogurt and avocado.

SERVES 6

Lycopene • 772mcg
Folate • 35%DV
Vitamin C • 132%DV

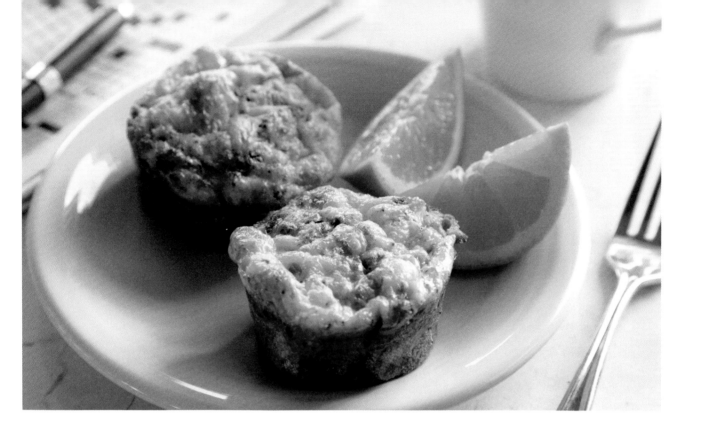

Broccoli & Quinoa Mini-Quiches

1¼ cups steamed broccoli, chopped

½ cup orange bell pepper, diced

½ cup cooked quinoa (page 166)

6 omega-3 eggs

¼ cup organic milk of choice

¼ tsp paprika, smoked or sweet

¼ tsp black pepper

¼ tsp sea salt

½ cup organic cheese (Parmesan, Romano or cheddar)

1. Preheat oven to 350°F. Place all ingredients except the cheese into a bowl; whisk to combine.

2. Spoon into lightly oiled unlined muffin cups. Sprinkle the tops of each quiche with cheese.

3. Bake for 15-20 minutes, until the center is risen and the eggs are set. A paring knife should come out clean. Serve while hot.

MAKES 9 MINI QUICHES

Can be made ahead and individually frozen. Microwave to reheat for a fast weekday morning breakfast.

Lutein+Zeaxanthin • 299mcg
Omega-3 • 179mg
Vitamin C • 36%DV

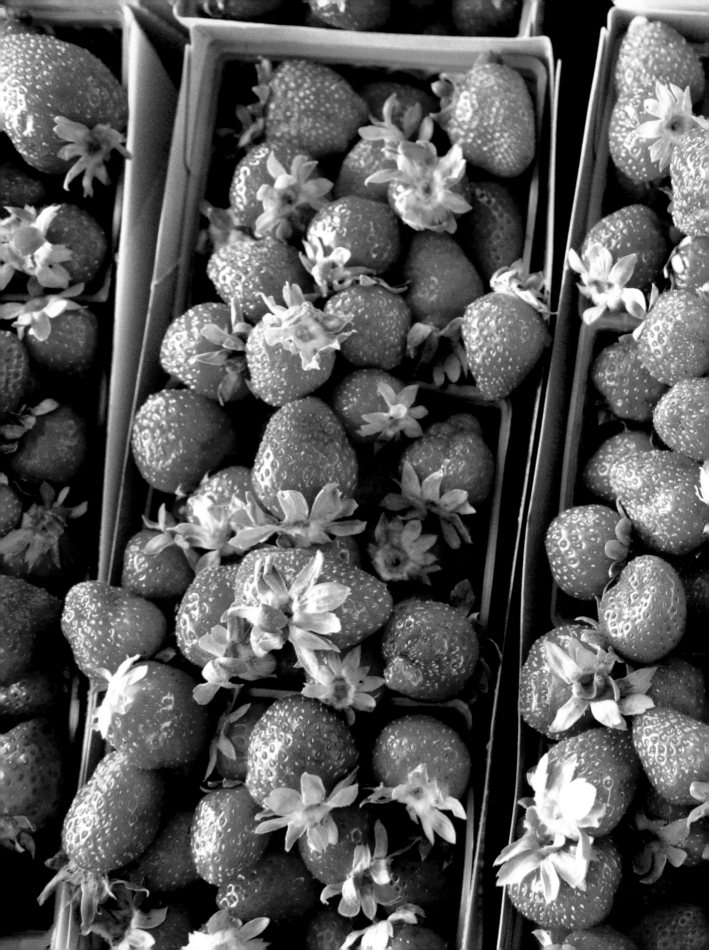

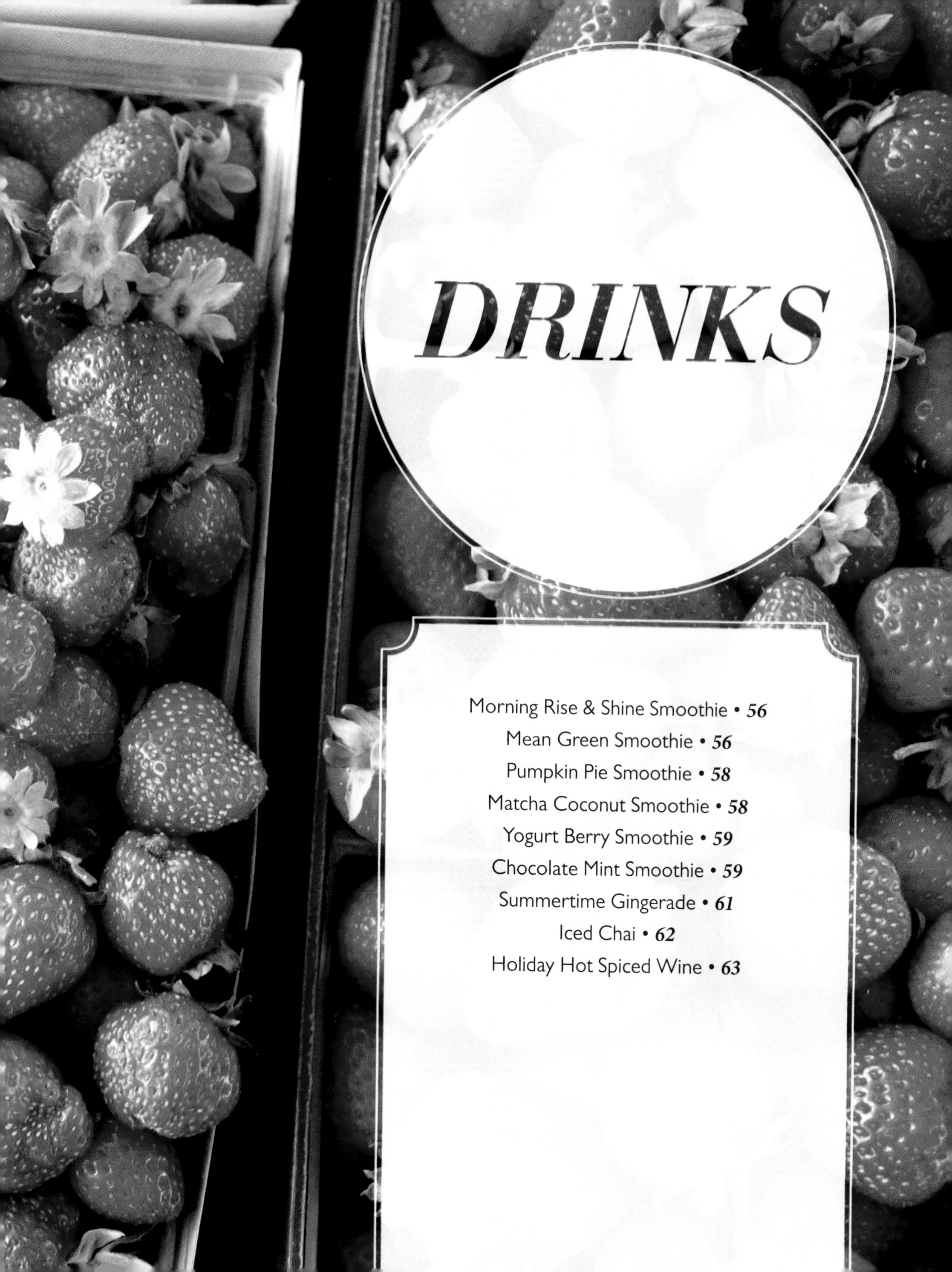

DRINKS

Morning Rise & Shine Smoothie • **56**

Mean Green Smoothie • **56**

Pumpkin Pie Smoothie • **58**

Matcha Coconut Smoothie • **58**

Yogurt Berry Smoothie • **59**

Chocolate Mint Smoothie • **59**

Summertime Gingerade • **61**

Iced Chai • **62**

Holiday Hot Spiced Wine • **63**

Smoothies

Add all ingredients to a blender. Puree until smooth. A high-speed blender works the best to create the "smoothest" of smoothies.

Morning Rise & Shine Smoothie   SERVES 2

- 1 kiwi, peeled
- ½ cup açaí juice
- ¼ cup frozen blueberries
- 1 Tbsp goldenberries
- 1 Tbsp chia seeds
- 1 scoop of your favorite protein powder
- 4 ice cubes

Vitamin A • 23%DV
Omega-3 • 1,204mg
Vitamin C • 115%DV

Mean Green Smoothie   SERVES 1

- ½ cup orange bell pepper
- ⅓ cup carrot, chopped
- 1 leaf raw kale, destemmed or 2 Tbsp cooked kale
- ⅓ cup cucumber, diced
- ½ banana
- 1½ tsp goji berries
- 1 scoop of your favorite protein powder
- 1½ tsp chia seed
- ½ cup organic unsweetened soymilk
- 4 ice cubes

Lutein+Zeaxanthin • 25,826mcg
Omega-3 • 1,557mg
Zinc • 16%DV

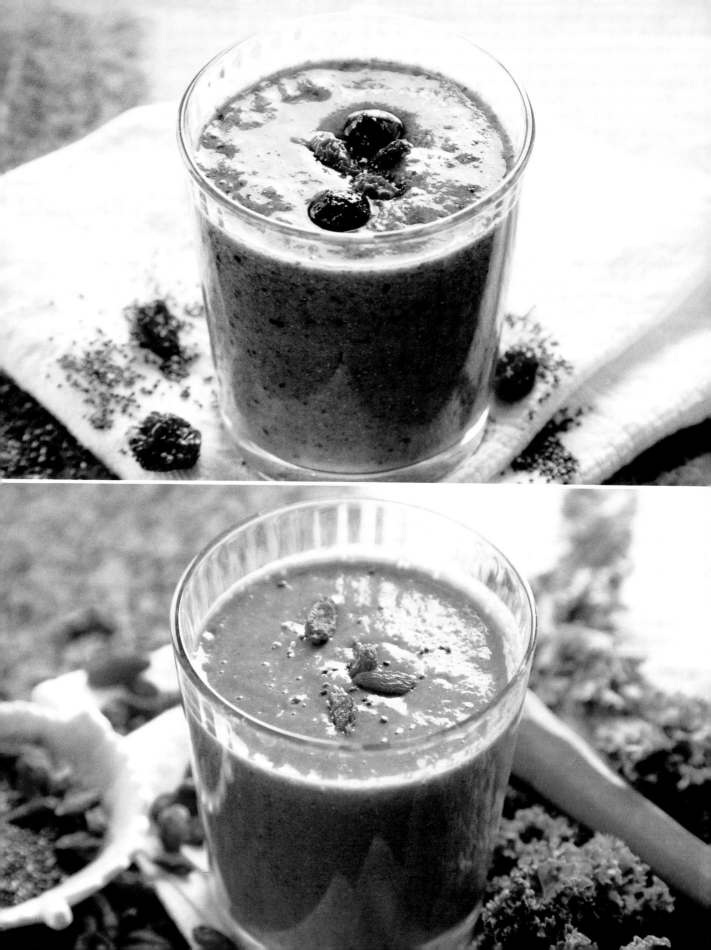

Pumpkin Pie Smoothie   SERVES 2

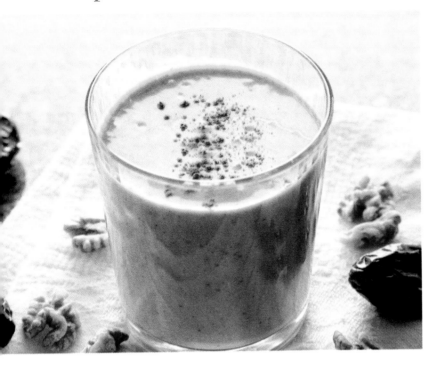

¼ cup pumpkin puree
¼ banana
2 medjool dates, pitted
¼ tsp cinnamon
¼ tsp powdered ginger
Pinch of nutmeg
Pinch of cloves
Pinch of allspice
1 Tbsp walnuts
2 Tbsp light coconut milk
½ cup unsweetened
   organic soy milk
1 scoop of your favorite
   protein powder
3 ice cubes

Beta-Carotene • 2,152mcg
Omega-3 • 372mg
Zinc • 7%DV

Matcha Coconut Smoothie   SERVES 2

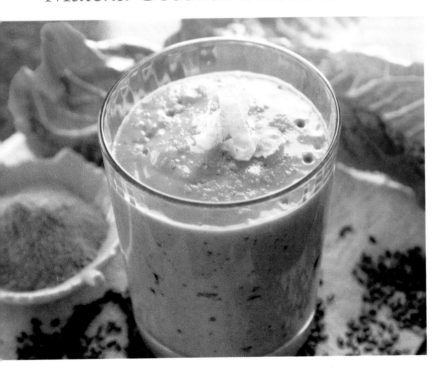

1½ tsp matcha powder
½ cup light coconut milk
1 cup romaine lettuce,
   roughly chopped
½ banana
½ avocado
2 medjool dates
1 Tbsp ground flax seed
¼ cup filtered water
1 scoop of your favorite
   protein powder
4 ice cubes

Lutein+Zeaxanthin • 670mcg
Omega-3 • 898mg
Folate • 25%DV

Yogurt Berry Smoothie

SERVES 2

½ cup plain Greek yogurt, non or low-fat
½ banana
1 cup frozen mixed berries
4 dried apricot halves
1 Tbsp ground flax seed
½ cup water
4 ice cubes

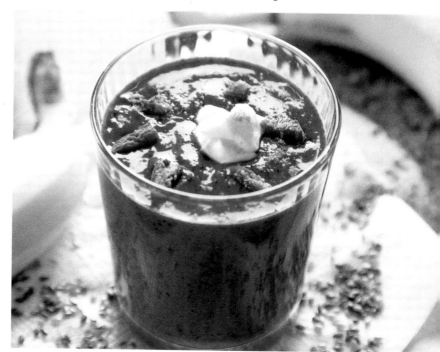

Beta-Carotene • 342mcg
Omega-3 • 1,725mg
Vitamin C • 84%DV

Chocolate Mint Smoothie

SERVES 2

¾ cup brewed peppermint tea, chilled
1 mint leaf
1 Tbsp cacao nibs
1 Tbsp natural cocoa powder
3 medjool dates, pitted
½ banana
1 Tbsp chia seeds
1 scoop of your favorite protein powder
6 ice cubes

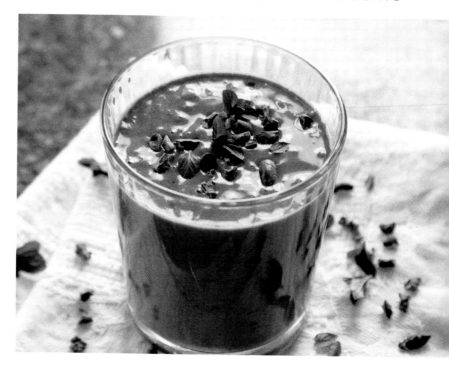

Omega-3 • 1,176mg
Vitamin B6 • 11%DV
Zinc • 9%DV

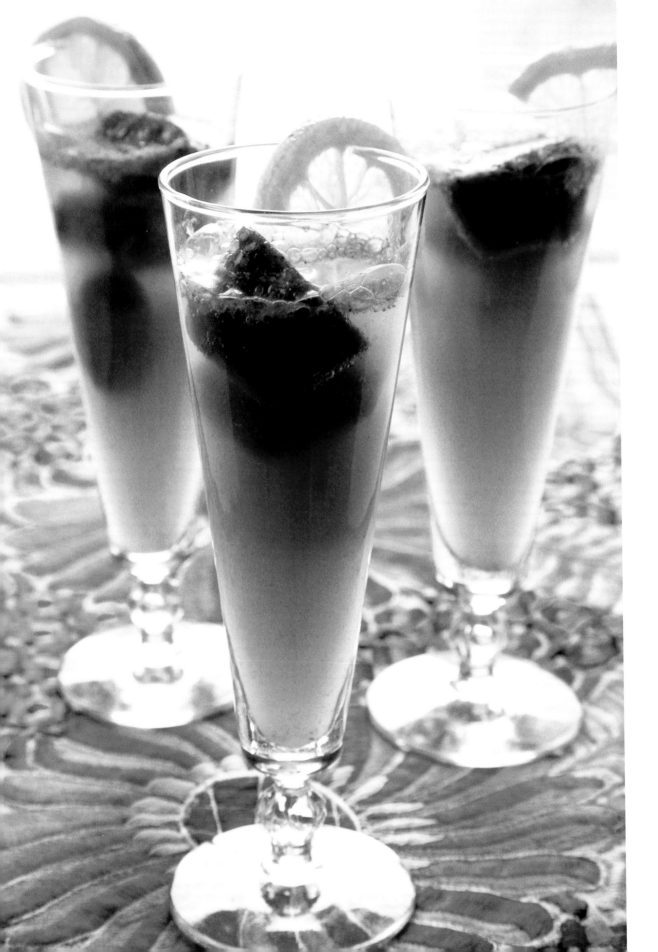

Summertime Gingerade

1 lb fresh ginger

2 cups seedless watermelon, cubed
1 cup blueberries
2 Tbsp lime juice
2 Tbsp chia seeds
   + ¼ cup water

2 Tbsp lime juice
3 Tbsp agave nectar

2 liters soda water

1. Using the edge of a spoon, peel the ginger. Rinse and pat dry. Freeze overnight, or longer if more convenient.

2. Whisk together chia seeds and ¼ cup water. Set aside for 15 minutes to hydrate.

3. For the watermelon berry ice cubes, puree the watermelon, blueberries, lime juice and hydrated chia seeds. Pour into ice cube trays. After freezing, remove from the tray and seal in a freezer bag until ready to use.

4. Allow the ginger to fully thaw to room temperature. To express the juice from the ginger, use a citrus press or crush between the handles of a pair of tongs.

5. Combine the ginger juice, lime juice and agave nectar.

6. To serve, add 3 tbsp of the ginger-lime mixture and 6 ounces soda water to a tumbler. Float 2-3 ice cubes. Garnish with fresh lime.

SERVES 6

Lycopene • 6,889mcg
Omega-3 • 2,328mg
Vitamin C • 57%DV

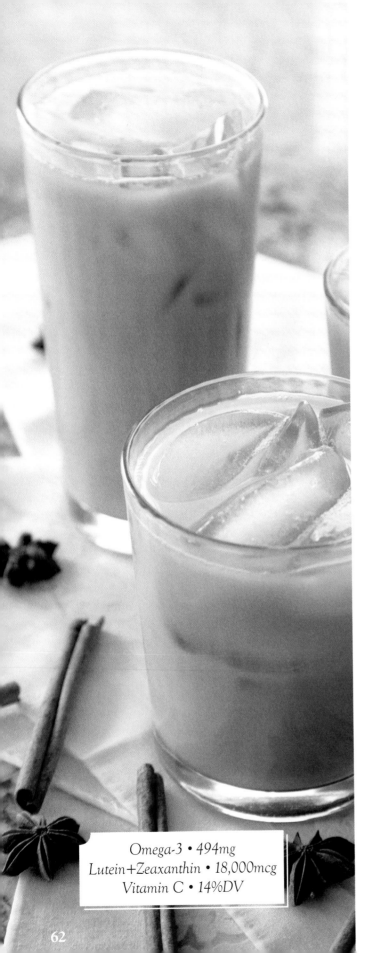

Iced Chai

2½ cups filtered water
3-4 black tea bags
½ tsp black pepper
½ tsp ground cardamom
1" piece fresh ginger, cut into coin-sized slices
4 whole star anise
4" cinnamon stick, broken into pieces
¾ cup organic unsweetened soymilk
1-2 Tbsp turbinado sugar, optional
½ cup ice cubes

1. Bring water to a boil in a sauce pan. Remove from heat and add the tea bags, ground pepper, cardamom, ginger, star anise and cinnamon stick.

2. Cover and steep for 15 minutes.

3. Strain through a fine mesh strainer.

4. Add the sugar and soy milk, stir to dissolve. Refrigerate until ready to use. Serve over ice.

MAKES 3¾ CUPS • SERVES 4

Omega-3 • 494mg
Lutein+Zeaxanthin • 18,000mcg
Vitamin C • 14%DV

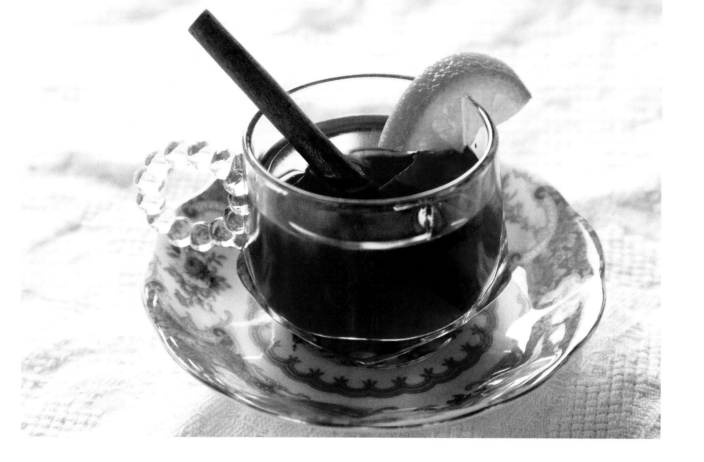

Holiday Hot Spiced Wine

4 cups brewed spiced tea, e.g.
  Constant Comment®
2 cups dry red wine
6 whole cloves
1 star anise
1 cinnamon stick
⅓ cup agave nectar

Cinnamon sticks and orange
  slices, for garnish

Slow-cooker, optional

Juice of half an orange
Half an orange, cut into slices

1. In a slow-cooker or sauce pan, combine the brewed tea and wine, along with the remaining ingredients.

2. The drink will be ready to serve when hot. Keep heated on low to serve as needed.

SERVES 8

Omega-3 • 30mg
Vitamin C • 11%DV

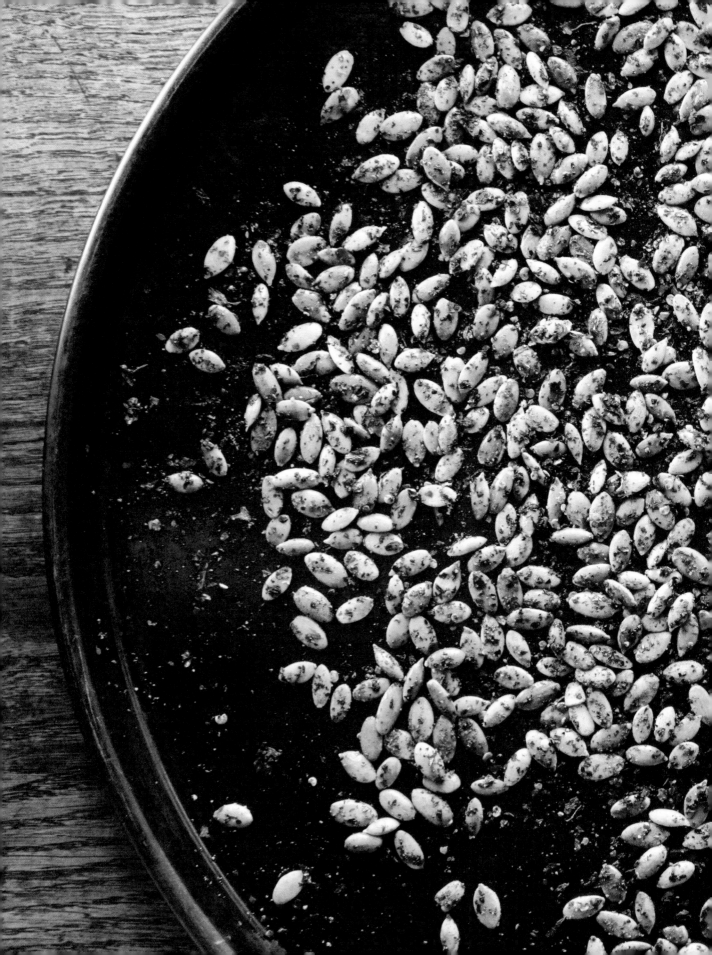

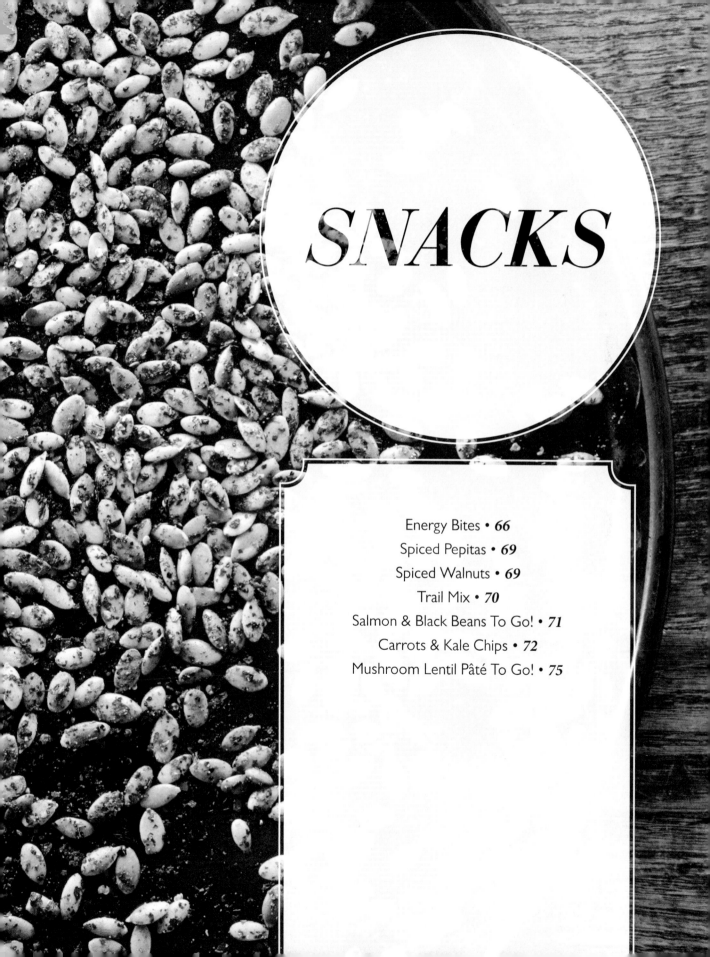

SNACKS

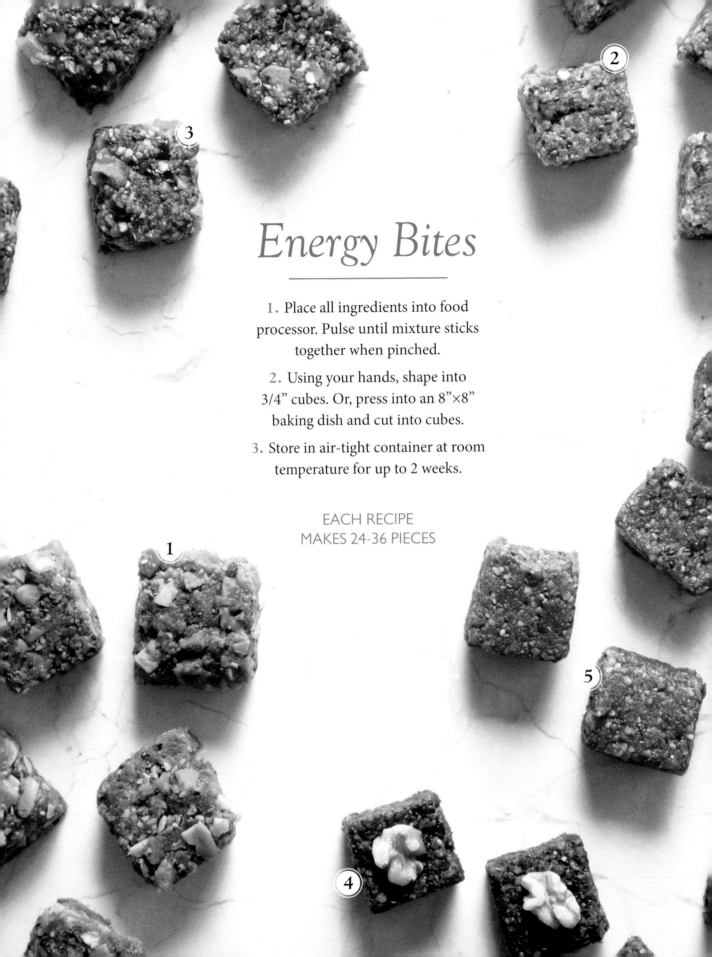

Energy Bites

1. Place all ingredients into food processor. Pulse until mixture sticks together when pinched.

2. Using your hands, shape into 3/4" cubes. Or, press into an 8"×8" baking dish and cut into cubes.

3. Store in air-tight container at room temperature for up to 2 weeks.

EACH RECIPE
MAKES 24-36 PIECES

1 Mexican Spice

- 1 cup walnuts
- 3 medjool dates, pitted
- 3 Tbsp ground flax seeds
- 1 Tbsp chia seeds
- 3 Tbsp unsweetened shredded coconut
- ½ cup mango pieces
- ⅓ cup pepita seeds
- ¼ tsp cayenne pepper
- ½ tsp ground turmeric
- ¼ cup protein powder
- 2 tsp lime juice
- 2 tsp water
- ⅛ tsp sea salt

Beta-Carotene • 42mcg
Omega-3 • 684mg
Zinc • 3%DV

2 Matcha & Ginger

- 1 cup walnuts
- 5 Turkish figs
- 2 Tbsp ground flax seeds
- 1 Tbsp chia seeds
- ¼ cup unsweetened shredded coconut
- 4 tsp matcha powder
- ¼ cup quinoa flakes
- 2 Tbsp protein powder
- 1 tsp ginger powder
- 1 tsp lemon zest
- 2 Tbsp lemon juice
- ⅛ tsp sea salt

Lutein+Zeaxanthin • 7mcg
Omega-3 • 614mg
Zinc • 2%DV

3 Mango, Cherry & Goji

- 1 cup walnuts
- 3 medjool dates, pitted
- 3 Tbsp ground flax seeds
- 1 Tbsp chia seeds
- 3 Tbsp unsweetened shredded coconut
- ⅓ cup protein powder
- 1½ Tbsp water
- ½ tsp almond extract
- 1 tsp vanilla extract
- ½ cup quinoa flakes
- ¼ cup goji berries
- ¼ cup dried tart cherries
- ¼ cup dried mango pieces

Lutein+Zeaxanthin • 2,060mcg
Omega-3 • 692mg
Zinc • 3%DV

4 Chocolate & Coffee

- 1 cup walnuts
- 4 medjool dates, pitted
- 2 Tbsp protein powder
- ¼ cup quinoa flakes
- 1 Tbsp chia seeds
- 2 Tbsp ground flax seeds
- ¼ cup unsweetened shredded coconut
- 2 Tbsp cacao nibs
- 2 Tbsp natural cocoa powder
- 1 Tbsp vanilla extract
- 2 Tbsp brewed coffee

Omega-3 • 624mg
Folate • 3%DV
Zinc • 2%DV

5 Apricot & Goji

- 1 cup walnuts
- 2 Tbsp ground flax seeds
- 1 Tbsp chia seeds
- 2 Tbsp protein powder
- ¼ cup quinoa flakes
- ¼ cup dried apricot
- ¼ cup goji berries
- 5 Turkish figs
- ⅛ tsp sea salt
- 1 Tbsp orange juice
- 1 tsp orange zest

Lutein+Zeaxanthin • 2,060mcg
Omega-3 • 547mg
Zinc • 2%DV

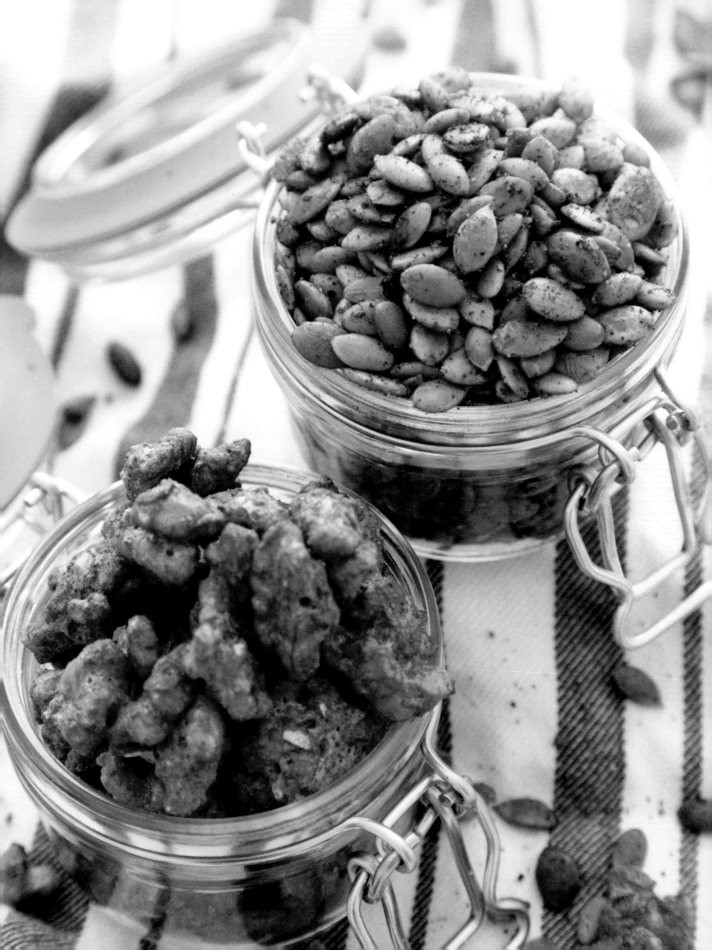

Spiced Pepitas

2 cups pepitas
2 tsp extra virgin olive oil
2 Tbsp of your favorite
  "Eye Spice" Blend,
  (pages 201-203)

1. Mix together and bake at 300°F for 8-12 minutes, stirring once or twice. Allow to cool before storing.

2. Store for up to 2 weeks in an airtight container.

MAKES 2 CUPS • SERVES 32

A delicious addition to your favorite dinner salad.

Beta-Carotene • 20mcg
Omega-3 • 19mg
Zinc • 4%DV

Spiced Walnuts

1 Tbsp grade B maple syrup
2 Tbsp water
1 egg white
2 cups walnuts, untoasted

1 Tbsp cinnamon
1 tsp ground ginger
¼ tsp nutmeg
¼ tsp allspice
¼ tsp white pepper
⅛ tsp sea salt
1 tsp arrowroot starch

1. Preheat oven to 250°F. To a bowl, add maple syrup, water and egg white. Beat lightly to combine. Add walnuts to the liquid ingredients, and let rest for 30 minutes, stirring once or twice.

2. In a separate bowl, stir together cinnamon, ginger, allspice, nutmeg, white pepper, salt and arrowroot starch.

3. Add spice mixture to soaked walnuts. Stir to evenly coat the walnuts. Spoon onto a parchment lined baking sheet.

4. Bake for 1 hour. Stir once or twice. Allow to cool thoroughly. Store in an airtight container for up to 2 weeks.

MAKES 2 CUPS • SERVES 8

Omega-3 • 2,271mg
Vitamin B6 • 7%DV
Zinc • 6%DV

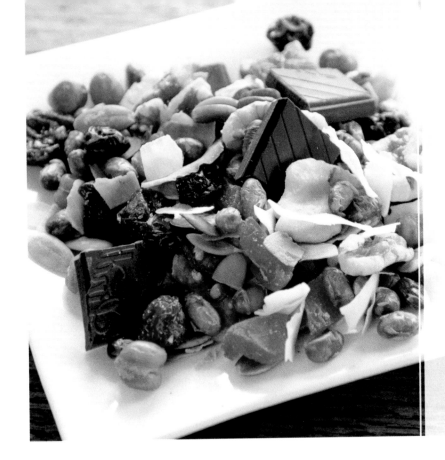

CHOOSE ONE OR MORE FROM EACH LIST BELOW:

nuts
pepitas, walnuts, pecans, almonds, soy nuts, macadamia nuts, brazil nuts, pistachios, chickpeas

dried fruit
cherries, blueberries, apricots, mango, cranberries, goldenberries, strawberries, goji berries

treats
unsweetened coconut flakes, dark chocolate chunks, toasted oats, whole wheat pretzels

Trail Mix

sample recipe

- 1 cup soy nuts
- 1 cup roasted chickpeas
- 1 cup walnuts
- ½ cup pepitas
- ½ cup dark chocolate chunks
- ½ cup toasted coconut flakes
- ¼ cup dried cherries
- ¼ cup apricots
- ¼ cup blueberries
- ¼ cup goldenberries

1. If using pre-roasted soy nuts, omit this step. Soak ½ cup raw soy nuts in filtered water for 6-8 hours or overnight. Rinse the soy nuts and place on a baking sheet.

2. Drain and rinse a can of chickpeas. Combine chickpeas and soaked soy nuts on a baking sheet. Roast for 1 hour and 20 minutes at 300°F, turning every 20 minutes for even roasting. Remove from oven and allow to cool for 20 minutes.

3. To create a personalized trail mix, combine desired ingredients from each list. Add the cooled soy nuts and roasted chickpeas.

4. Stir to combine. Store sealed at room temperature for up to 2 months.

MAKES 5½ CUPS •
SERVES 17

Omega-3 • 701mg
Folate • 11%DV
Zinc • 10%DV

Salmon & Black Beans To Go!

½ lb wild salmon,
   poached and flaked
   OR
2 cans (5 oz each)
   wild salmon,
   drained and flaked

15 oz can black beans,
   drained and rinsed
1 garlic clove, minced
2 Tbsp scallions, minced

2 Tbsp organic celery,
   finely minced
1 Roma tomato, finely diced
½ lime, juiced
¼ tsp sea salt
¼ tsp black pepper
1 jalapeño, finely minced,
   ribs and seeds removed,
   optional
3 Tbsp parsley or cilantro,
   roughly chopped

Lycopene • 585mcg
Omega-3 • 1,518mg
Folate • 31%DV

1. In mixing bowl, coarsely mash the black beans with a fork or pastry blender, leaving some whole.

2. Add garlic, scallions, celery, tomato, lime juice, salt, pepper and jalapeño, if using.

3. Gently stir in salmon to incorporate.

4. Garnish with parsley. Chill until ready to serve.

MAKES 2½ CUPS • SERVES 4

Serve with vegetable crudités or whole wheat pita for an easy and portable lunch.

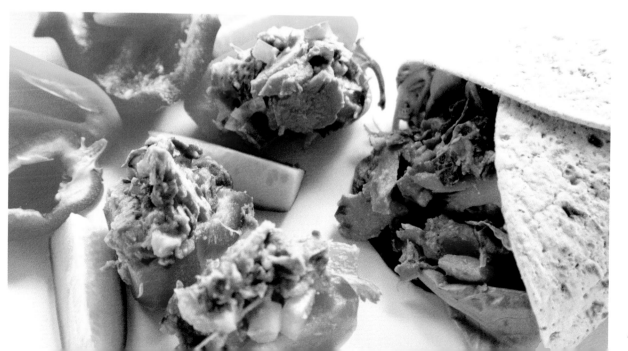

Carrots & Kale Chips

2 small carrots,
   coarsely chopped
½ cup raw pepita seeds
2 Tbsp lemon juice
⅔ cup water
2 Tbsp extra virgin olive oil
¼ tsp black pepper
½ tsp ground chipotle,
   optional
½ tsp garlic powder
½ tsp onion powder
1 tsp smoked paprika
1 tsp turmeric
2 Tbsp ground flax seed
½ tsp sea salt

2 bunches green curly
   kale, destemmed

High speed blender

1. Preheat oven to 275°F. Place all ingredients except kale into a high speed blender or food processor. Blend until smooth.

2. In a large mixing bowl, tear kale into chip-sized pieces. Pour the carrot mixture over the kale. Using your hands, massage the carrot mixture into the kale. Place onto one to two cookie sheets, as needed, lined with parchment paper.

3. Bake until the kale is dry and crispy, approximately 1½ hours, flipping every 30 minutes. Allow to cool in oven with door ajar for 30 minutes.

SERVES 6

To use a regular blender, steam the carrots until soft, and soak pepitas in ½ cup water for 30 minutes, drain.

Lutein+Zeaxanthin • 44,287mcg
Omega-3 • 794mg
Vitamin C • 232%DV

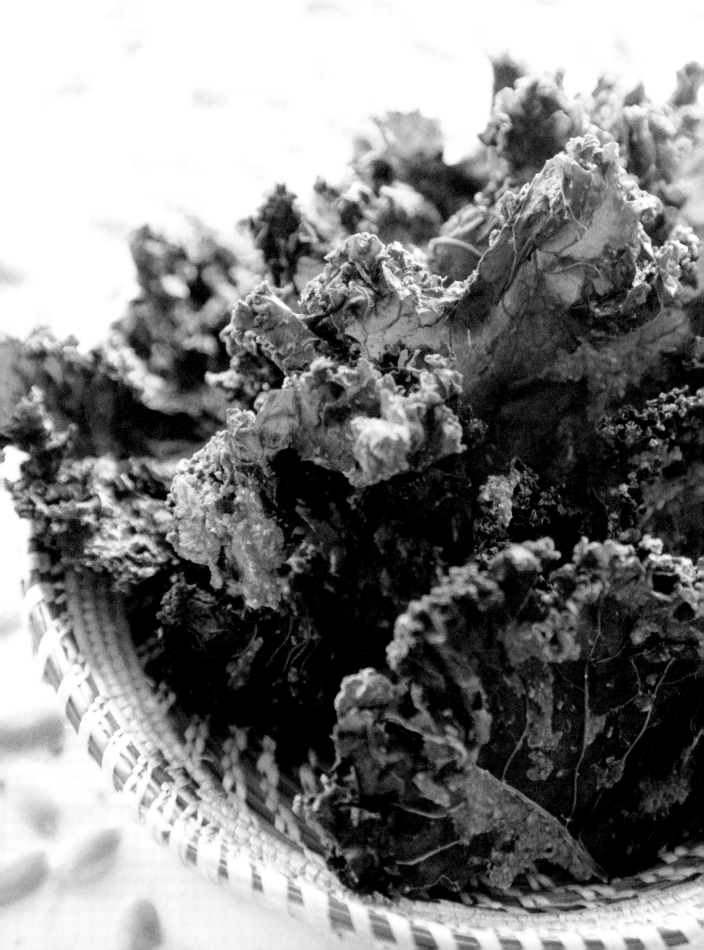

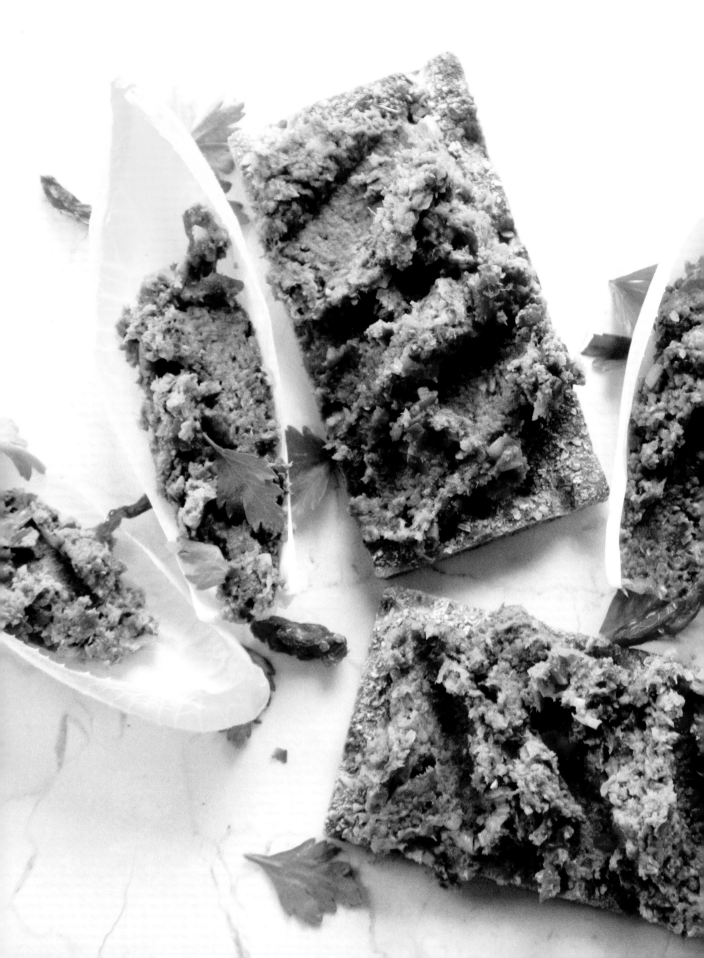

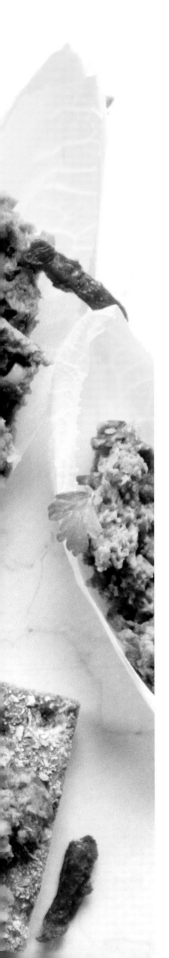

Mushroom Lentil Pâté To Go!

1 large onion,
   coarsely chopped
1 Tbsp extra virgin olive oil
1 garlic clove, minced
8 oz crimini mushrooms,
   sliced
1 cup cooked lentils
4 oz sardines, with bones
   and skin, drained
1 tsp paprika,
   smoked or sweet
1 Tbsp lemon juice
½ tsp lemon zest
¼ tsp sea salt
¼ tsp black pepper
½ tsp red pepper
   flakes, optional
¼ cup sun dried tomatoes,
¼ dried or packed in oil,
   drained and roughly
   chopped
2 cup Italian flat leaf parsley
1/2 cup scallions, diced

Belgian endives
Whole wheat high-fiber
   crackers

1. Preheat a skillet to medium, add the oil quickly followed by the onions. Sauté until onions are lightly caramelized, 6-8 minutes.

2. Add garlic and mushrooms to the onions. Sauté for 3-5 minutes until the juice from the mushrooms is mostly evaporated.

3. To a food processor, add mushroom-onion mixture, lentils, sardines, paprika, lemon juice, lemon zest, salt, black pepper and red pepper flakes, if using. Puree until smooth. Add sun dried tomatoes. Pulse to combine. Add parsley and scallions. Pulse 2-3 more times.

4. Serve with high-fiber crackers and whole endive leaves.

MAKES 3½ CUPS • SERVES 6

Lycopene • 2,060mcg
Omega-3 • 310mg
Vitamin B12 • 28%DV

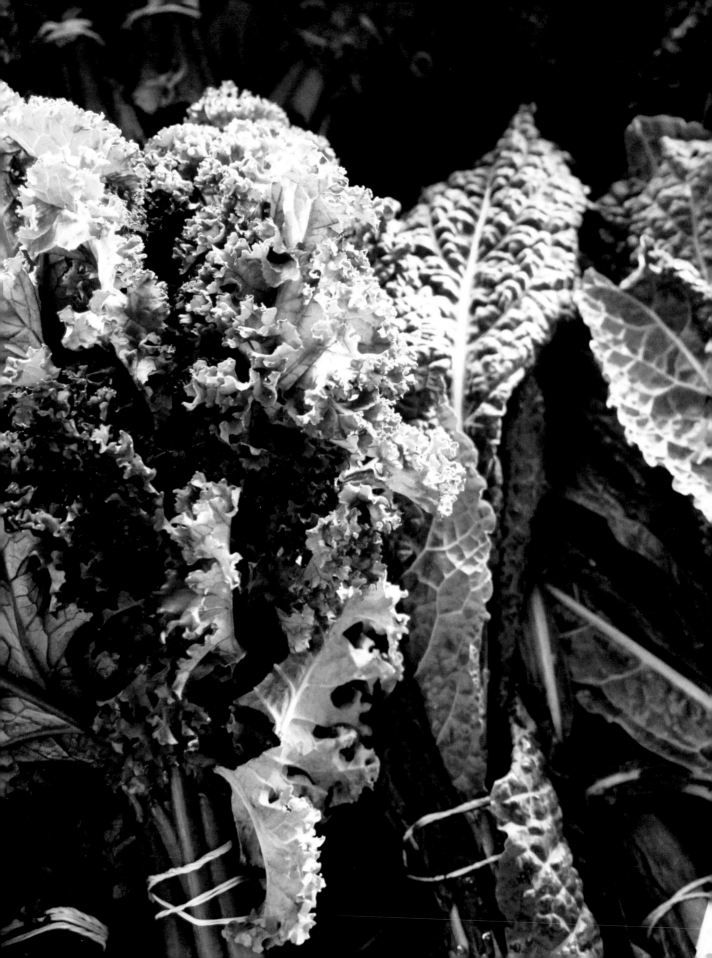

SALADS

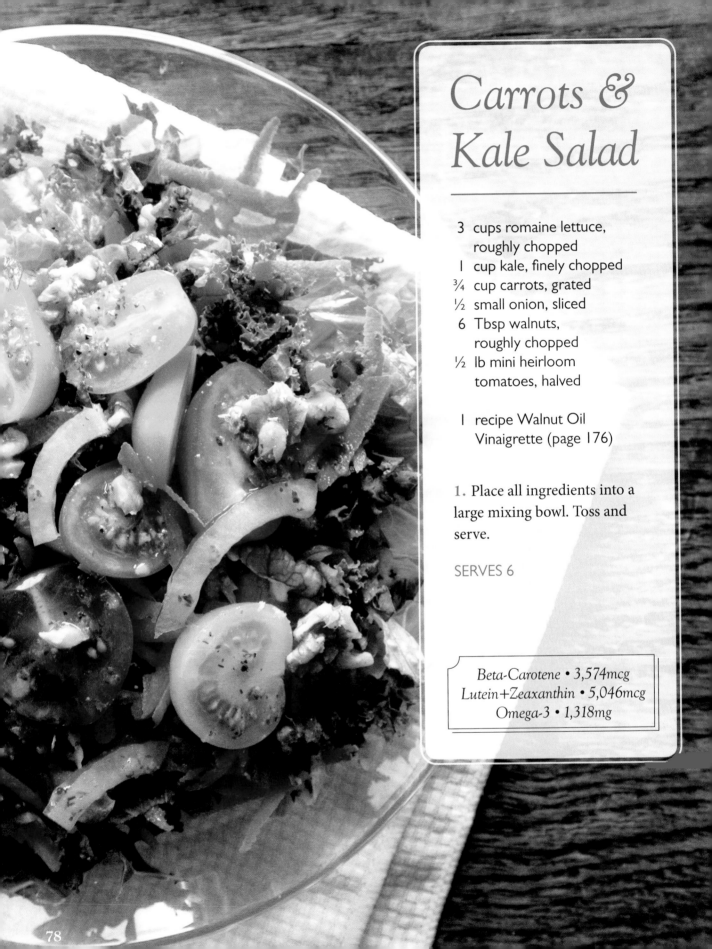

Carrots & Kale Salad

3 cups romaine lettuce, roughly chopped
1 cup kale, finely chopped
¾ cup carrots, grated
½ small onion, sliced
6 Tbsp walnuts, roughly chopped
½ lb mini heirloom tomatoes, halved

1 recipe Walnut Oil Vinaigrette (page 176)

1. Place all ingredients into a large mixing bowl. Toss and serve.

SERVES 6

Beta-Carotene • 3,574mcg
Lutein+Zeaxanthin • 5,046mcg
Omega-3 • 1,318mg

Avocado & Salmon Salad

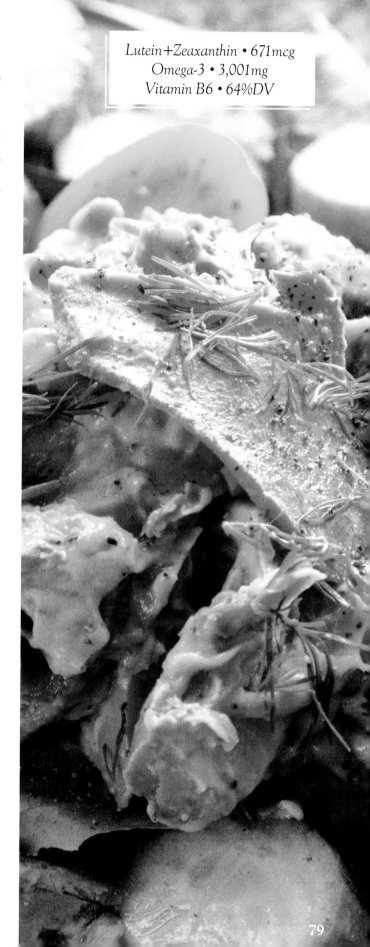

1 lb wild Alaskan salmon, cooked and flaked
OR
3 cans (5 oz each) wild salmon,
drained and flaked

1 avocado
2 Tbsp apple cider vinegar
2 Tbsp extra virgin olive oil
2 tsp fresh dill, minced
¼ tsp sea salt
¼ tsp black pepper
⅛ tsp cayenne, optional

2 tsp capers, chopped and rinsed if salted
¼ cup red onion, finely minced
⅓ cup celery, finely diced
1-2 Tbsp filtered water, to thin as needed

4 cups spring mix greens
4 radishes, sliced
2 Persian or hothouse cucumbers, sliced
1 cup mini heirloom tomatoes, halved

1. To a food processor add avocado, vinegar, olive oil, dill, salt, pepper and cayenne, if using. Puree until smooth. Transfer from food processor into a mixing bowl.

2. Stir in the capers, onion, celery and salmon. Thin with water, if needed, 1 Tbsp at a time.

3. Divide greens, radishes, cucumbers and tomatoes equally among 4 plates. Spoon avocado salmon salad equally over the greens and serve.

SERVES 4

Southwestern Salad

1¼ cups black beans,
    drained and rinsed
1 cup frozen corn, thawed
1 orange bell pepper, small dice
1 small jalapeño, ribs and seeds
    removed, small dice
1 vine-ripened tomato, small dice
1 small red onion, small dice
2 Tbsp parsley, minced
2 Tbsp cilantro, minced
1 garlic clove, finely minced
¼ tsp sea salt
½ tsp black pepper

1 recipe Achiote Lime Vinaigrette
   (page 176)

1. To a mixing bowl add black beans, corn, bell pepper, jalapeño, tomato, onion, parsley, cilantro, garlic, salt and pepper.

2. Stir in Achiote Lime Vinaigrette. Refrigerate until ready to serve.

MAKES 6½ CUPS • SERVES 10

This is a great recipe to share with your friends and family at your next picnic!

Lutein+Zeaxanthin • 169mcg
Folate • 13%DV
Vitamin C • 45%DV

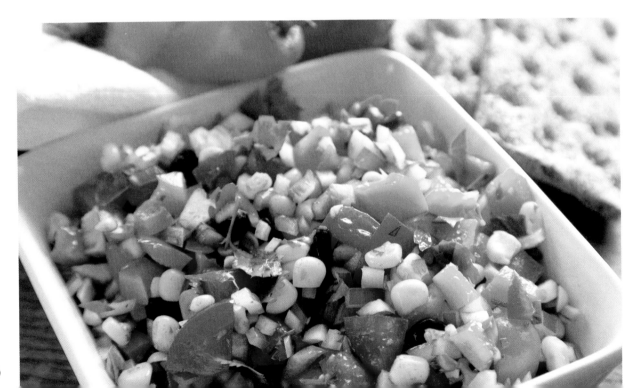

80

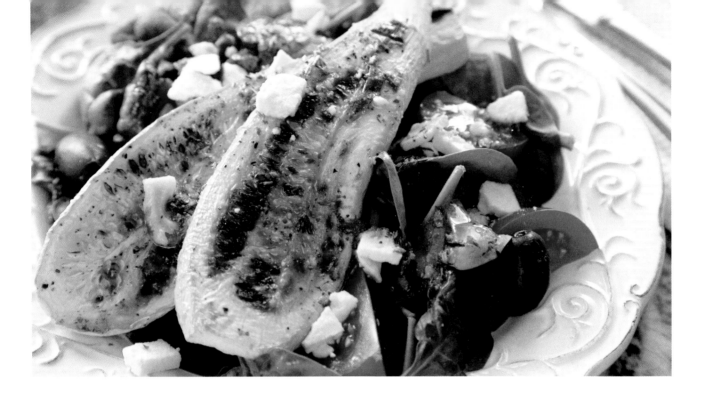

Roasted Summer Squash Salad

4 summer squash, sliced lengthwise, ½"
1 Tbsp extra virgin olive oil
⅛ tsp sea salt
¼ tsp black pepper

8 oz fresh spinach
6 oz feta cheese
24 kalamata olives
½ red or sweet onion, thinly shaved slices
6 Tbsp walnuts or pepita seeds
18 cherry tomatoes

1 recipe Walnut Oil Vinaigrette (page 176)

1. Preheat oven to 375°F. Place summer squash slices on a baking sheet. Drizzle with oil and sprinkle with salt and pepper. Bake for about 15 minutes until squash is soft and has taken on a little color. Remove from the oven.

2. Divide spinach between 6 plates. Lay the roasted summer squash on top.

3. Garnish with the feta, olives, onion, walnuts, and tomatoes. Spoon 1½ Tbsp walnut oil dressing on each salad.

SERVES 6

Lutein+Zeaxanthin • 7,426mcg
Omega-3 • 1,483mg
Zinc • 12%DV

Sesame Cucumber "Noodle" Salad

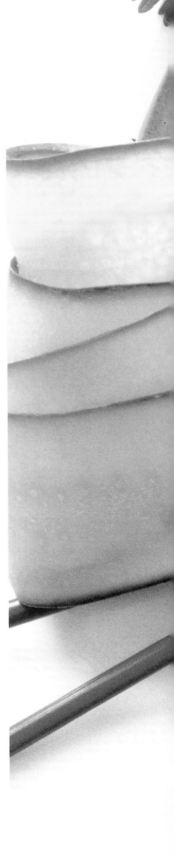

1 bunch asparagus spears
10 shiitake mushrooms, caps only, coarsely chopped
2 tsp extra virgin olive oil
2 Tbsp filtered water

2 large English cucumbers or 6 Persian/hothouse cucumbers, sliced into ribbons
1 cup seaweed salad, store-bought
1 recipe Asian Miso Dressing (page 186)

1 Tbsp black sesame seeds,
1 lightly roasted large sheet nori, crumbled

1. Peel the fibrous lower portion of the asparagus. Cut into bite-sized pieces.

2. Preheat heavy lidded skillet to medium high. Add the oil quickly followed by the asparagus and mushrooms. Stir constantly for 2 minutes. Turn off the heat, add the water and cover to steam for 5 minutes. The asparagus should be crisp-tender.

3. Divide cucumber "noodles" equally among 4 plates. Garnish each dish with seaweed salad, mushroom caps and asparagus.

4. Serve with Asian Miso Dressing. Sprinkle with sesame seeds and nori.

SERVES 4

Consider serving with a salmon fillet or Easy Smoked Salmon Sushi (page 133).

> *Lutein+Zeaxanthin • 861mcg*
> *Folate • 30%DV*
> *Vitamin E • 20%DV*

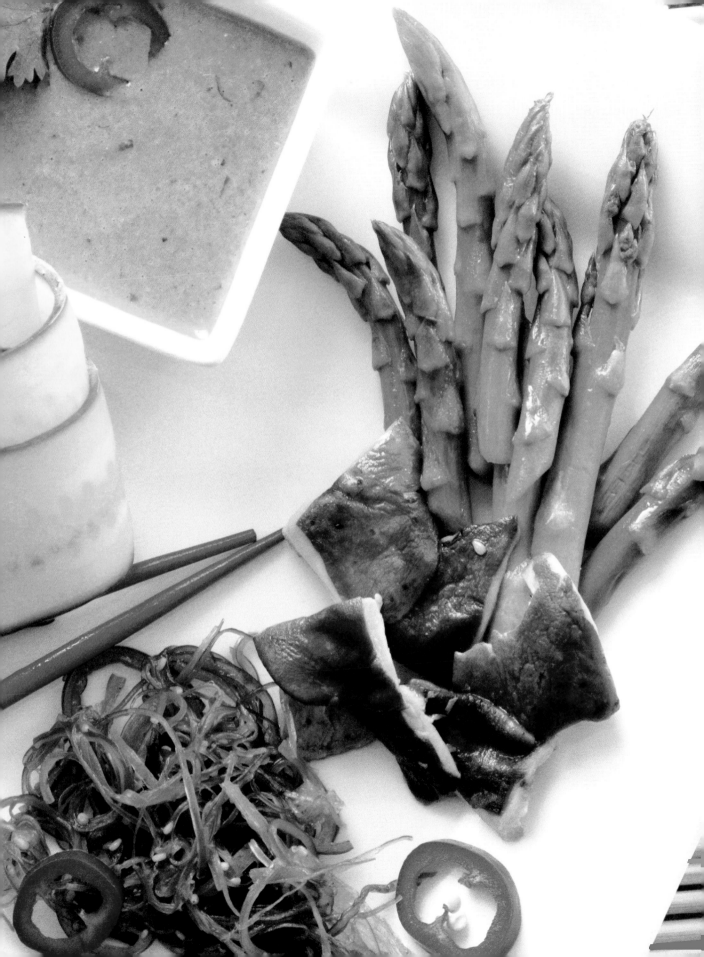

Rainbow Coleslaw

2 cups red cabbage, shredded

2 cups green cabbage, shredded

2 cups carrots, grated

½ cup Cumin Jalapeño Dressing (page 183)

1. Place all ingredients into a mixing bowl. Stir to combine and serve.

SERVES 6

This salad is a crowd pleaser!

Beta-Carotene • 3,214mcg
Vitamin B6 • 7%DV
Vitamin C • 48%DV

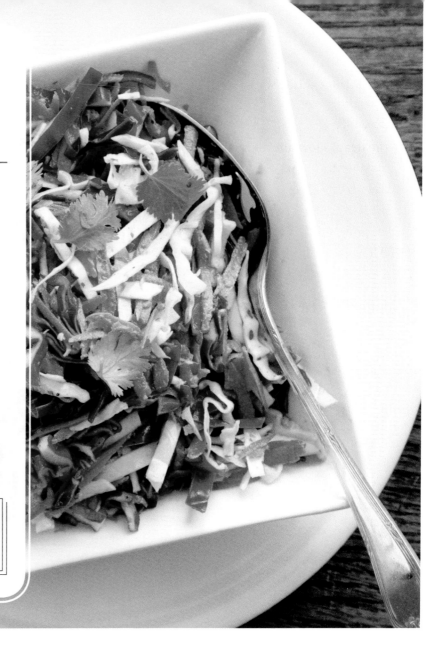

Sprouted Layer Salad recipe continued on next page ›››

1 cup dried sprouted beans, e.g., mung beans, green lentils, and adzuki, such as TruRoots® brand

3 cups filtered water

½ cup Cumin Jalapeño Dressing, divided (page 183)

2 cups corn, frozen

2 cups orange bell pepper, ½" dice

1 Tbsp chipotle in adobo

¼ tsp sea salt

2 avocados, diced

1 small red onion, small dice

1 jalapeño, ribs and seeds removed, minced

1 lime, juiced

⅓ cup cilantro, chopped

12 oz cherry tomatoes, halved

1. For the bean layer, add water and the beans to a sauce pan, bring to a boil over medium heat. Reduce the heat to low and cover. Simmer for 5 minutes. Remove from the heat and allow to steep, covered, for 10 minutes. Drain, if needed. Allow to cool.

2. Stir in ¼ cup cumin jalapeño dressing.

3. For the corn and bell pepper layer, combine corn and bell pepper with chipotle in adobo and salt. Stir.

4. For the avocado jalapeño layer, combine avocados, red onion, jalapeño, lime juice, pinch of salt and cilantro in a small mixing bowl. Stir.

5. To assemble, place beans in the bottom of a serving bowl. Add the corn and bell pepper layer, followed by avocado layer. Top with halved tomatoes. Pour final ¼ cup dressing over the top. Refrigerate 1 hour before serving.

SERVES 10

Lutein+Zeaxanthin • 335mcg
Vitamin C • 92%DV
Vitamin E • 8%DV

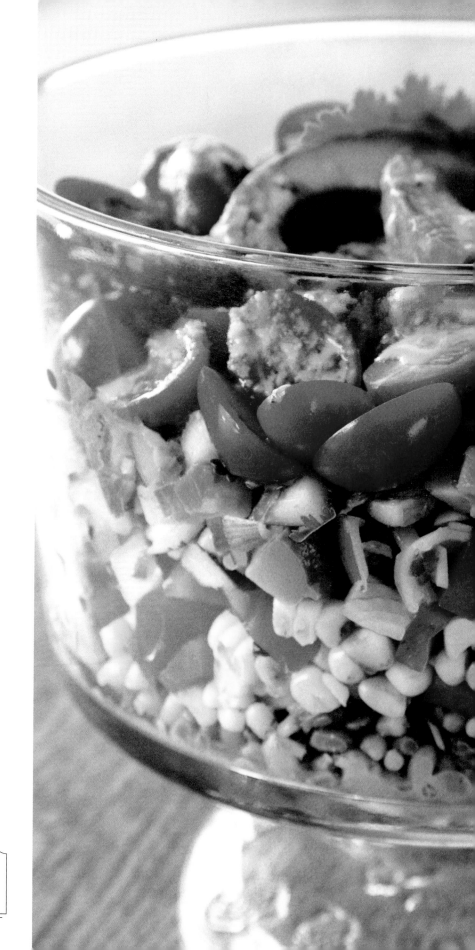

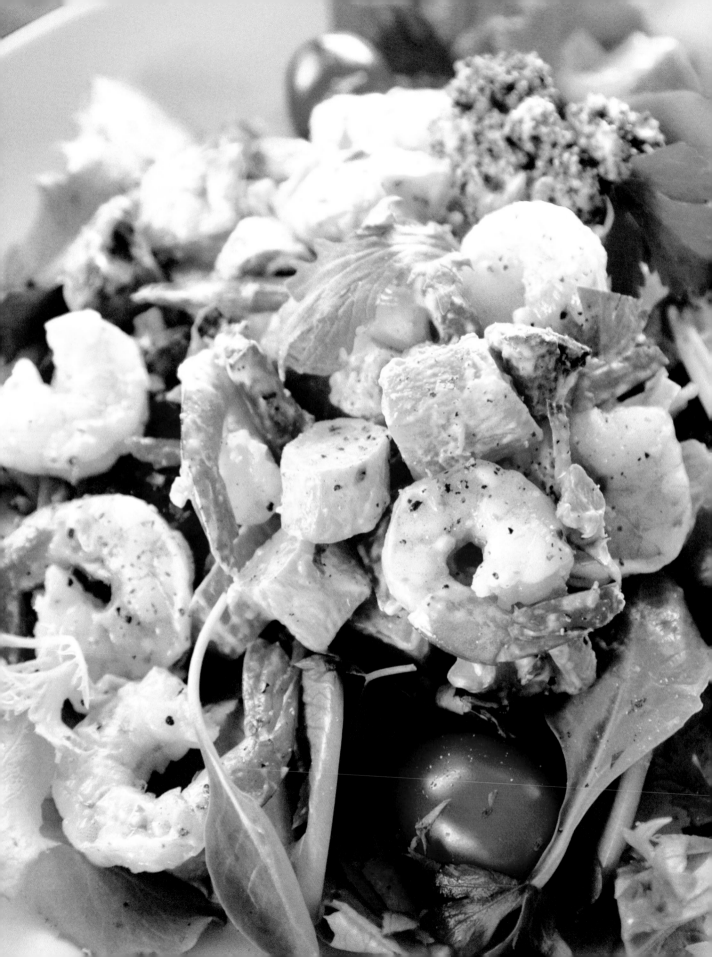

Shrimp & Roasted Vegetable Salad with Goat Cheese Dressing

3 cups butternut squash, cut into ½" pieces
2 cups broccoli florets, cut into bite-sized pieces
3 cups cauliflower florets, cut into bite-sized pieces
2 cups red and orange bell peppers, cut into bite-sized pieces
8 oz crimini mushrooms, quartered (2½ cups)
1 sweet onion, coarsely chopped
¼ tsp sea salt
½ tsp black pepper
3 Tbsp extra virgin olive oil

8 oz spring mix greens
¾ cup parsley, chopped
2 Persian cucumbers, sliced
1 carrot, shredded
1 cup cherry tomatoes
1 lb shrimp, cooked, peeled and deveined

⅔ cup Avocado Goat Cheese Dressing (page 177)

1. Preheat oven to 375°F. In a large mixing bowl combine butternut squash, broccoli, cauliflower, bell pepper, mushrooms and onion. Sprinkle with salt and pepper, drizzle with olive oil, and stir to evenly coat.

2. Pour onto a baking sheet and roast for 20-30 minutes, until crisp tender, stirring twice. Remove from oven and allow to cool for 15 minutes.

3. For the salad, combine spring mix lettuce, parsley, cucumbers, carrot, tomatoes and shrimp. Divide among 6 plates, top with roasted vegetables, and drizzle with dressing. Serve immediately.

SERVES 6

Wild poached salmon or wild canned salmon would be a healthful substitute for the shrimp. This recipe can easily be cut in half. To simplify, only use 1 or 2 of the vegetables to roast.

Lutein+Zeaxanthin • 1,778mcg
Omega-3 • 402mg
Vitamin C • 262%DV

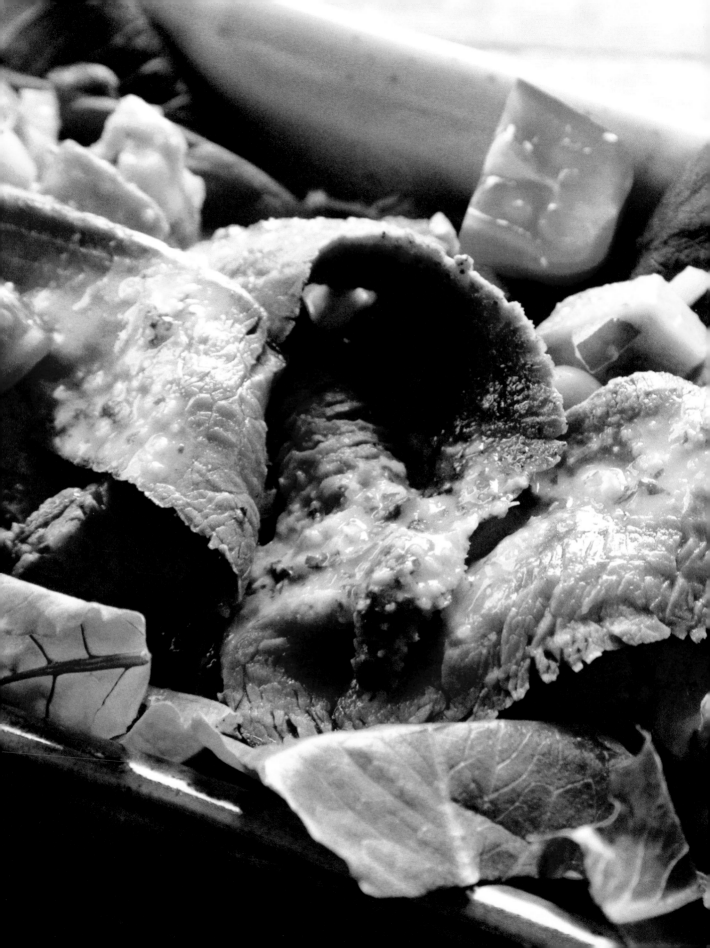

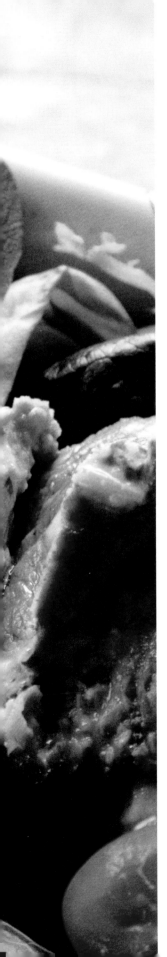

Steak Salad with Cumin Jalapeño Vinaigrette

4 cups spring mix greens

⅓ cup red onion, finely diced
1 large heirloom tomato,
  cut into wedges
1 avocado, diced
¾ cup corn kernels,
  fresh or frozen
¾ cup black beans, cooked
2 Tbsp Cumin Jalapeño
  Vinaigrette (page 183)

1 lb grass-fed flank
  or skirt steak
¼ tsp sea salt
¼ tsp black pepper
1 Tbsp extra virgin olive oil

⅓ cup Cumin Jalapeño
  Vinaigrette (page 183)

1. Divide the spring mix equally among 4 plates.

2. In a small bowl combine onion, tomato, avocado, corn and black beans. Drizzle with 2 Tbsp vinaigrette. Allow to marinate while grilling steak.

3. Preheat a skillet to medium high. Sprinkle steak with salt and pepper. Pour oil into the skillet quickly followed by the steak. Allow to cook 4-5 minutes. Turn over, and cook 4-5 more minutes. Remove from heat, cover and allow to rest 5-10 minutes before slicing. For medium, the internal temperature should read 140-145°F.

4. Spoon marinated vegetable mixture equally over spring mix. Slice steak and divide equally. Serve with extra dressing.

SERVES 4

Lutein+Zeaxanthin • 761mcg
Vitamin B6 • 49%DV
Zinc • 48%DV

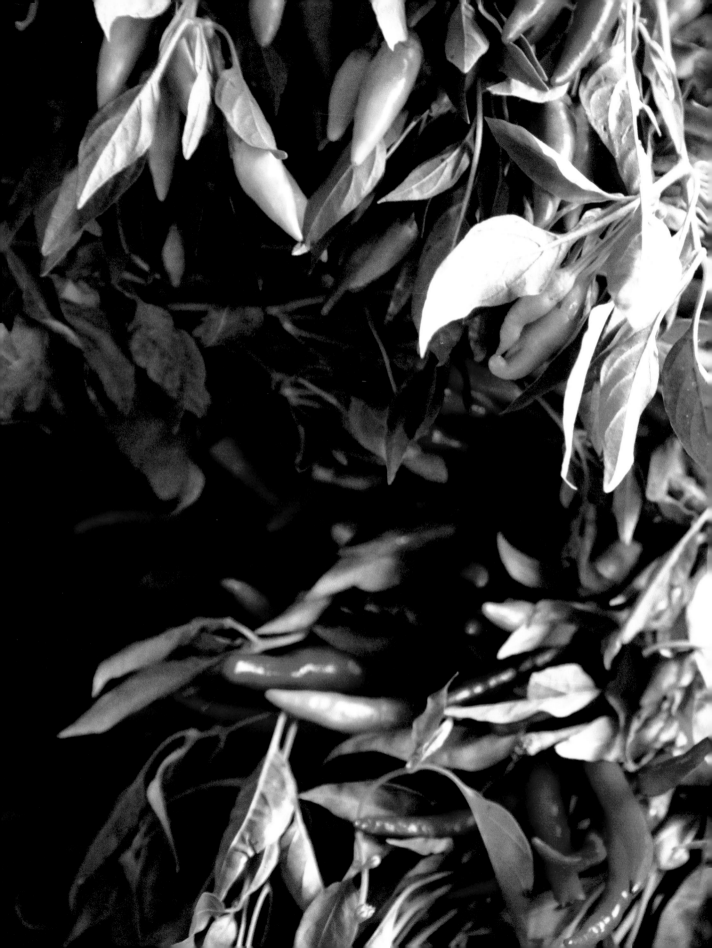

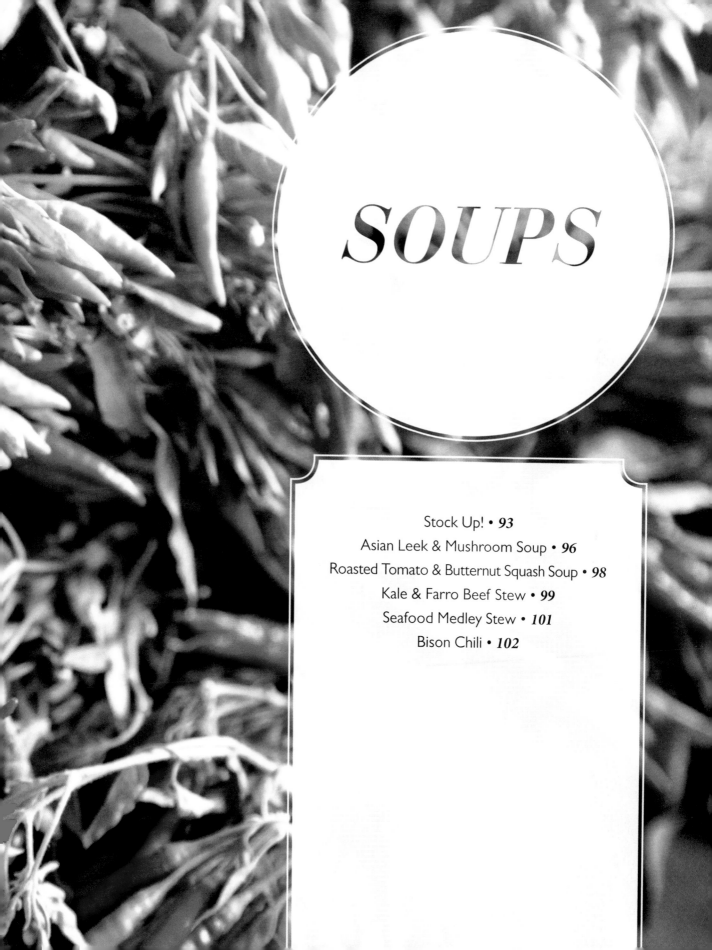

SOUPS

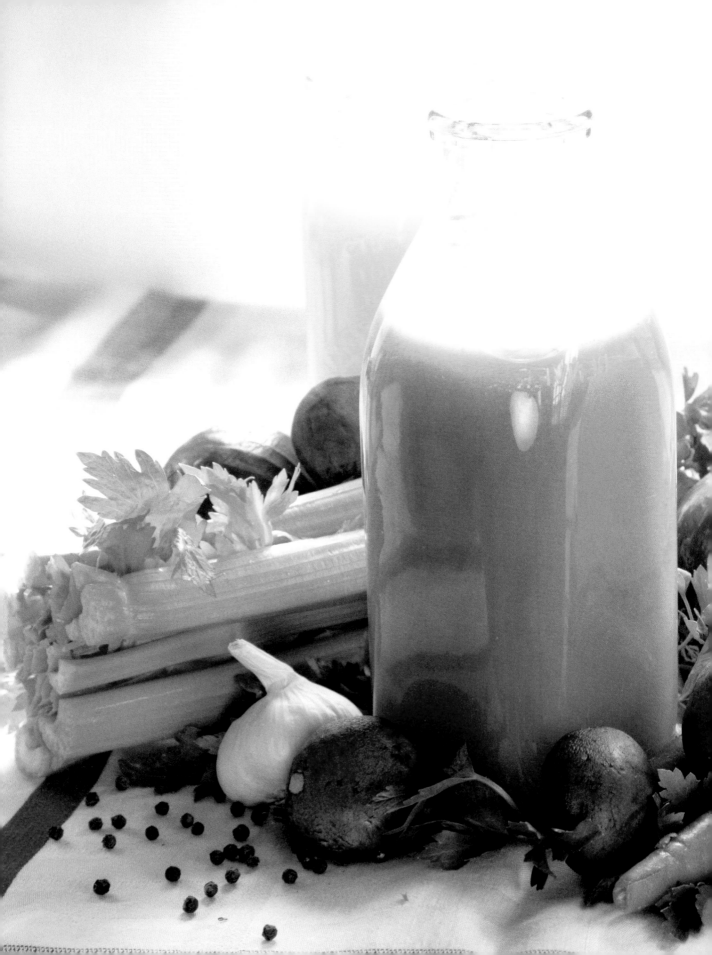

Stock Up!

Stocks have great nutrition and flavor. Make in advance and freeze in a variety of convenient sizes available at a moments notice.

- Well made stocks are low calorie and rich in vitamins, minerals and protein.

- The protein in stock is a delicious way to help regulate blood glucose.

- Mineral extraction from the bones is enhanced by the addition of an acid such as vinegar or lemon juice.

- Vitamin retention is aided by using a lid and by adding the vegetables towards the end of the cooking process.

- Use an ice bath to chill the stock efficiently. Stocks should always be cooled as quickly as possible to avoid spoilage.

- Store stocks refrigerated 2-3 days or frozen up to 3 months.

- For convenience, defat stocks prior to freezing.

- To increase the nutrient profile, substitute stock for water when cooking grains, soups and vegetables.

- Stock vs. Broth: Stock is an ingredient ready to use in a recipe. Broth is a completed seasoned soup.

VEGETABLE STOCK
Lycopene • 791mcg
Lutein+Zeaxanthin • 967mcg
Vitamin C • 25%DV

POULTRY STOCK
Omega-3 • 247mg
Vitamin B6 • 25%DV
Zinc • 14%DV

FISH STOCK
Lutein+Zeaxanthin • 491mcg
Omega-3 • 1,125mg
Vitamin B12 • 89%DV

BEEF STOCK
Lutein+Zeaxanthin • 301mcg
Omega-3 • 228mg
Zinc • 26%DV

recipes continued on next page ›››

Vegetable

3 cups chopped vegetables of choice
5 cups water

OR

1 Tbsp extra virgin olive oil
1 small leek, roughly sliced
2 garlic cloves, mashed
1 carrot, roughly diced
2 ribs celery with leaves, roughly chopped
1 tomato, coarsely diced
1 cup romaine lettuce, roughly chopped
⅓ bunch parsley
½ cup mushrooms
½ tsp whole black peppercorns
6 cups filtered water

1. To a 4½ qt or larger stock pot, preheated to medium, add oil quickly followed by the leek and garlic. Sauté until softened, 3-5 minutes.

2. Add the remaining ingredients with enough water to cover the vegetables. Slowly bring to a boil, then reduce the heat to low. Cover and simmer for 1 hour. Remove from the heat and allow to cool, covered. Strain through a fine mesh.

3. Refrigerate and use within 3 days or freeze in convenient sized portions.

MAKES 1 QUART

Fish

1 Tbsp extra virgin olive oil
½ medium onion or leek, chopped
1 carrot, chopped
1 rib celery, chopped
1 garlic clove, mashed
5 cups filtered water
2 Tbsp lemon juice
½ tsp whole black peppercorns
4 sprigs fresh parsley
1½ lb fish trimmings (heads minus the gills, bones, tails)

1. To a 4½ quart or larger stock pot preheated to medium, add the oil quickly followed by the onions, carrots, celery and garlic. Sauté 3-4 minutes. Add water, lemon juice, peppercorns, parsley and fish trimmings.

2. Cover and simmer on low for 20 minutes. Remove any accumulated scum. Remove from heat and allow to cool, covered, for 20 minutes.

3. Strain through a fine mesh. Refrigerate and use within 2 days or freeze immediately in convenient sized portions.

This fish stock recipe can be used in Seafood Medley Stew (page 101).

MAKES 1 QUART

Poultry

4 lb poultry (backs, necks, wings,
    carcass from a roasted bird)
4 quarts cold water,
    or more as needed
2 Tbsp vinegar
1 small leek or onion,
    coarsely chopped
1 medium carrot,
    coarsely chopped
1 rib celery, coarsely chopped
¼ cup dried shiitake mushrooms
    or 4 oz fresh mushrooms
½ bunch parsley
2 sprigs thyme
2 garlic cloves, mashed
1 tsp whole black peppercorns

1. In a 7 qt or larger stock pot, add the poultry, water and vinegar. Water should cover the bones by 1 inch; add more water, if necessary. Slowly bring to a boil and reduce heat to a simmer, uncovered for 30 minutes. Remove any scum that accumulates.

2. Partially cover the stockpot and simmer on low for 3 hours.

3. Add onion, carrot, celery, mushrooms, parsley, thyme, garlic and peppercorns. Cover and simmer over low heat 1 hour.

4. Remove from heat and allow to cool, covered, for 30 minutes.

5. Strain and refrigerate immediately. When thoroughly chilled, remove the solidified fat. Refrigerate and use within 2 days or freeze in convenient sized portions.

MAKES 2 QUARTS

Beef

6 lb lean beef bones (shin, neck,
    marrow, shank, or rib bones)
4 quarts cold water
3 Tbsp vinegar
1 small onion or leek, large dice
2 carrots, large dice
2 Tbsp tomato paste
4 oz mushrooms
3 garlic cloves, mashed
1 bay leaf
1 tsp whole black peppercorns
1 cup celery,
    including leaves, diced
½ bunch of parsley

1. Preheat oven to 375°F. In a 7 qt or larger stockpot, roast the bones until they are brown, about 40-50 minutes. Remove from the oven and place on the stove top.

2. Add 4 quarts of water or more to cover the bones by at least 1". Add the vinegar.

3. Slowly bring the uncovered stock to a boil, then reduce to a simmer for 30 minutes. Remove any scum that accumulates.

4. Partially cover and simmer on low for 6-8 hours.

5. Add onions, carrots, tomato paste, mushrooms, garlic, bay leaf, peppercorns, celery and parsley. Cover and simmer for 1 hour. Allow to cool, covered, 30 minutes.

6. Strain and refrigerate immediately. When thoroughly chilled, remove the solidified fat. Refrigerate and use within 2 days or freeze in convenient sized portions.

MAKES 2 QUARTS

Asian Leek & Mushroom Soup

1 Tbsp extra virgin olive oil
1½ cups leeks, white and light green parts only, sliced and thoroughly washed
2 garlic cloves, finely minced
1 Tbsp fresh ginger, grated

1½ cups shiitake mushrooms, destemmed and sliced
4½ cups high-quality stock of choice
1 Tbsp soy sauce or tamari
6 oz firm tofu, ½" cubes
3 scallions, sliced
3 Tbsp cilantro, roughly chopped

1. To a large stock pot preheated to medium, add the olive oil quickly followed by the leeks, garlic and ginger. Sauté 1-2 minutes.

2. Add the mushrooms and stock. Bring up to a simmer for one minute. Add the soy sauce and tofu. Simmer an additional minute.

3. Garnish with the scallions and cilantro. Serve hot.

SERVES 6

Consider serving as a first course to your favorite stir-fry.

Lutein+Zeaxanthin • 516mcg
Vitamin B6 • 10%DV
Zinc • 5%DV

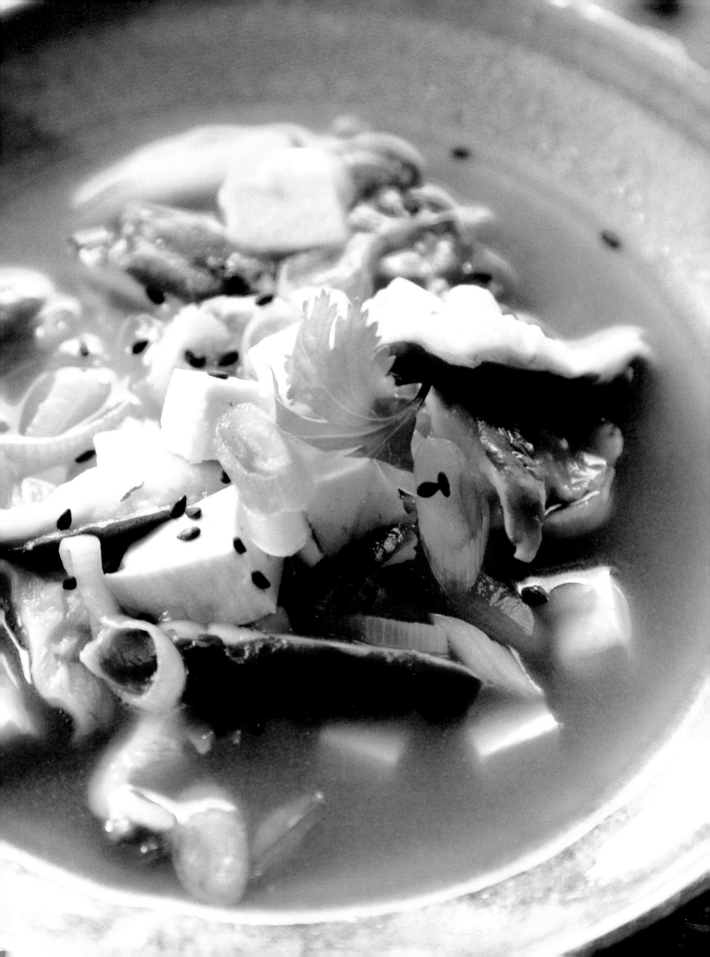

Roasted Tomato & Butternut Squash Soup

1 ½ lb Roma tomatoes,
    halved length-wise
2 tsp extra virgin olive oil
¼ tsp sea salt

1 ½ lb butternut squash,
    halved and seeded
    (about 2 ½ cups cubed)
1 tsp extra virgin olive oil

1 sweet onion,
    roughly chopped
1 Tbsp extra virgin olive oil
2 garlic cloves, minced
½ tsp sea salt

3 cups homemade
    chicken stock, defatted

1. Preheat oven to 325°F. Place Roma tomatoes cut side up into an oven safe glass baking dish. Drizzle with olive oil and sprinkle with ¼ tsp sea salt. Roast for 1 hour 15 minutes until lightly caramelized.

2. Rub the cut-side of the butternut squash with olive oil. Place the squash cut-side down on a baking sheet. Roast for 1 hour until lightly caramelized.

3. In a heavy skillet preheated to medium-high, add olive oil quickly followed by the onion, garlic and salt. Sauté for 5-8 minutes or until softened and beginning to take on color. Remove from the heat.

4. Puree all ingredients with chicken stock until smooth. Return to the pot to heat through.

SERVES 4

Use caution when blending hot ingredients. Place kitchen towel over blender lid for safety. Consider serving with Parsley Basil Pesto (page 196) and grated Parmesan.

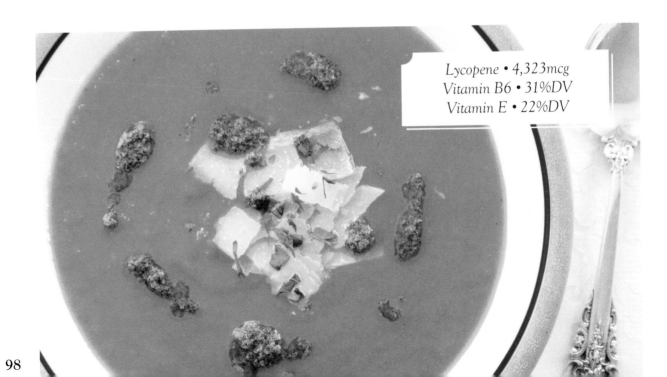

Lycopene • 4,323mcg
Vitamin B6 • 31%DV
Vitamin E • 22%DV

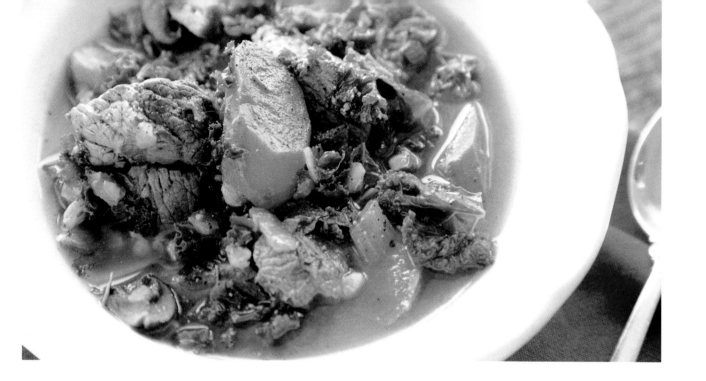

Kale & Farro Beef Stew

1 ¼ lb London broil steak, ½" cubes

2 Tbsp extra virgin olive oil, divided

¼ tsp sea salt

2 garlic cloves, minced

½ sweet onion, diced

4 cups filtered water or stock of choice

2 tsp bouquet garni

1 bay leaf

¼ tsp sea salt

¼ tsp black pepper

¾ cup carrots, diced

4 oz crimini mushrooms, quartered

⅓ cup pearled farro, uncooked

¾ cup kale, finely chopped

1. Preheat a large Dutch oven to medium-high heat. Sprinkle meat with sea salt. Add 1 Tbsp oil quickly followed by the meat. Brown the meat very well, about 10-15 minutes. Remove the meat from the pot and set aside.

2. Add 1 Tbsp olive oil to the same pot along with the garlic and onions. Sauté 2-3 minutes.

3. Add water or stock, browned meat, bouquet garni, bay leaf, salt and pepper. Bring up to a boil, reduce the heat to low. Cover and simmer for 45 minutes until beef is nearly tender.

4. Add carrots, mushrooms and farro. Cover and simmer for 20 minutes. Add the kale, simmer for another 10 minutes. Serve hot.

MAKES 2 ½ QUARTS • SERVES 7

Lutein+Zeaxanthin • 2,876mcg
Vitamin B12 • 48%DV
Zinc • 25%DV

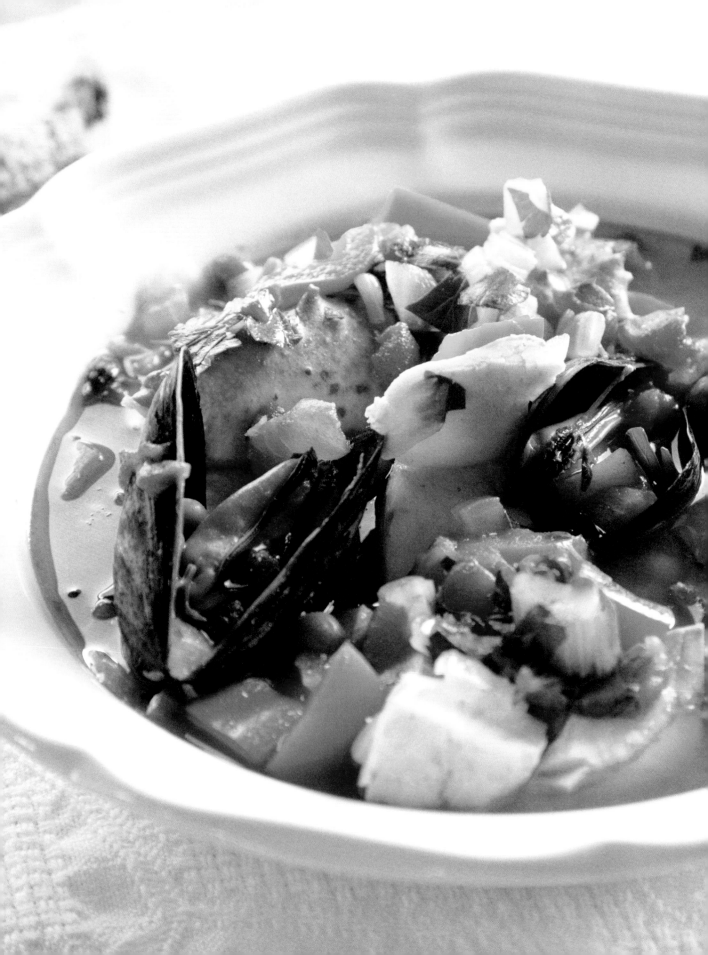

Seafood Medley Stew

1 Tbsp extra virgin olive oil
1 large onion, diced
3 garlic cloves, sliced
¾ cup celery, diced
1 orange bell pepper, diced
14.5 oz can petite diced tomatoes

6 cups chicken stock
OR
3 cups fish stock +
3 cups water

1 bay leaf
1 tsp smoked paprika
1 sprig rosemary
¼ tsp red pepper flakes
½ tsp black pepper

1 lb mussels, scrubbed and debearded
1 lb extra large raw shrimp, deveined, peeled or unpeeled
¾ lb tilapia, cut into 1" chunks
¾ lb Alaskan king crab, cut into 4" pieces
1½ cups baby peas, frozen
⅓ cup Italian flat leaf parsley, roughly chopped

1. To a large Dutch oven preheated to medium, add oil quickly followed by onion, garlic, celery and bell pepper. Sauté until vegetables soften, about 5 minutes.

2. Add diced tomatoes and continue to cook an additional 3 minutes, stirring occasionally.

3. Add the stock, bay leaf, paprika, rosemary, red and black pepper. Cover and bring to a simmer for 15 minutes. The stew may be made ahead of time up to this point. Refrigerate until needed.

4. Return to a simmer, if made ahead. Remove the bay leaf. Add the mussels. Cover and simmer for 3 minutes.

5. Add the raw shrimp and tilapia. Cover and continue to simmer an additional 3 minutes.

6. Finally add the crab and peas. Simmer 1-2 minutes.

7. Keep the stew covered until ready to serve. Garnish with parsley. Serve hot with whole grain rice.

MAKES 3½ QUARTS • SERVES 8

The quality of the stew is all about the quality of the ingredients, most notably the seafood and stock. This recipe can easily be cut in half. Although there are a lot of ingredients in this stew, cooking time is less than 30 minutes.

Lutein+Zeaxanthin • 985mcg
Omega-3 • 735mg
Zinc • 32%DV

Bison Chili

2 Tbsp extra virgin olive oil, divided
1¼ lb ground bison

3 garlic cloves, minced
1 large red onion, small dice
2 ribs celery, small dice
1 orange bell pepper, small dice
6 oz can tomato paste
14 oz can organic diced tomatoes
4 oz can green chilies
2 Tbsp cacao nibs, ground
15 oz can black beans, drained and rinsed
½ tsp ground cumin
1 tsp sea salt
½ tsp black pepper

1 Tbsp dried oregano
2 Tbsp mild chili powder
1 Tbsp chipotle in adobo, optional
4 cups filtered water or stock of choice
1 cup frozen corn

Diced cilantro, tomatoes and onions, for garnish

1. Preheat a large Dutch oven to medium-high. Add 1 Tbsp olive oil quickly followed by the bison and a pinch of salt and pepper. Sauté to lightly brown the meat. Remove the meat and reserve.

2. To the same pot, add remaining olive oil followed by the garlic, onion, celery and bell pepper. Sauté until softened, about 5 minutes, scraping the pan to release the brown bits.

3. Add the tomato paste and sauté 4-5 minutes, stirring frequently.

4. Add the green chilies, cacao nibs, black beans, cumin, salt, black pepper, oregano, chili powder, chipotle, if using, water or stock, and reserved bison. Cover and simmer on low for 1½ - 2 hours.

5. Just before serving, stir in the frozen corn and allow to come to temperature.

MAKES 3 QUARTS • SERVES 8

Lycopene • 7,397mcg
Vitamin B6 • 27%DV
Zinc • 27%DV

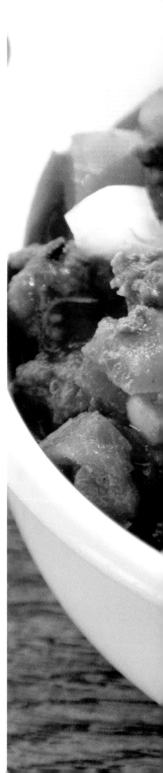

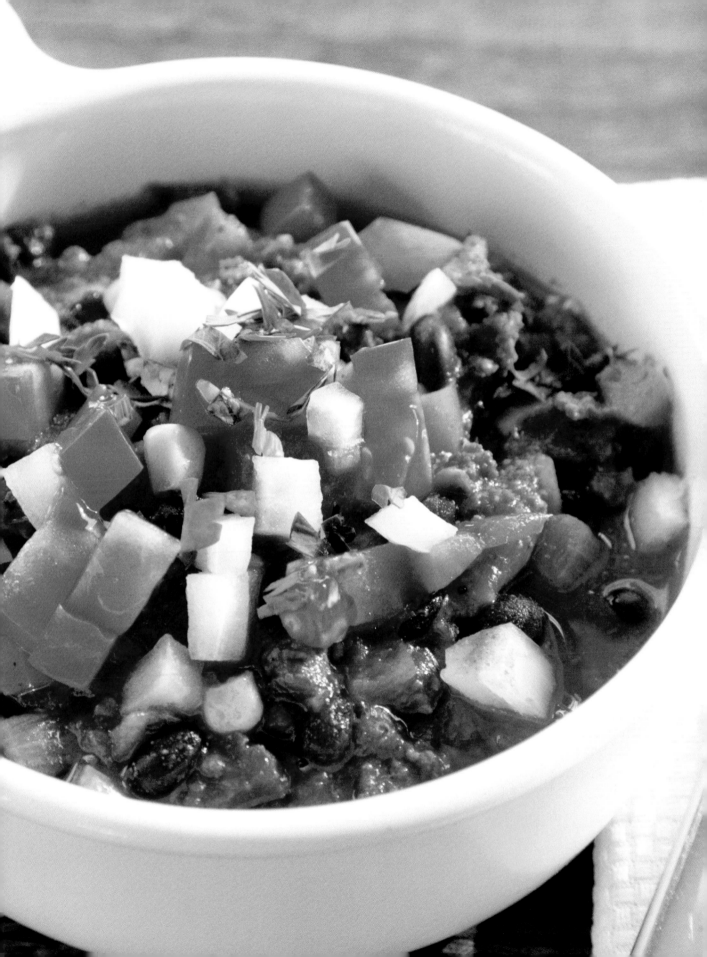

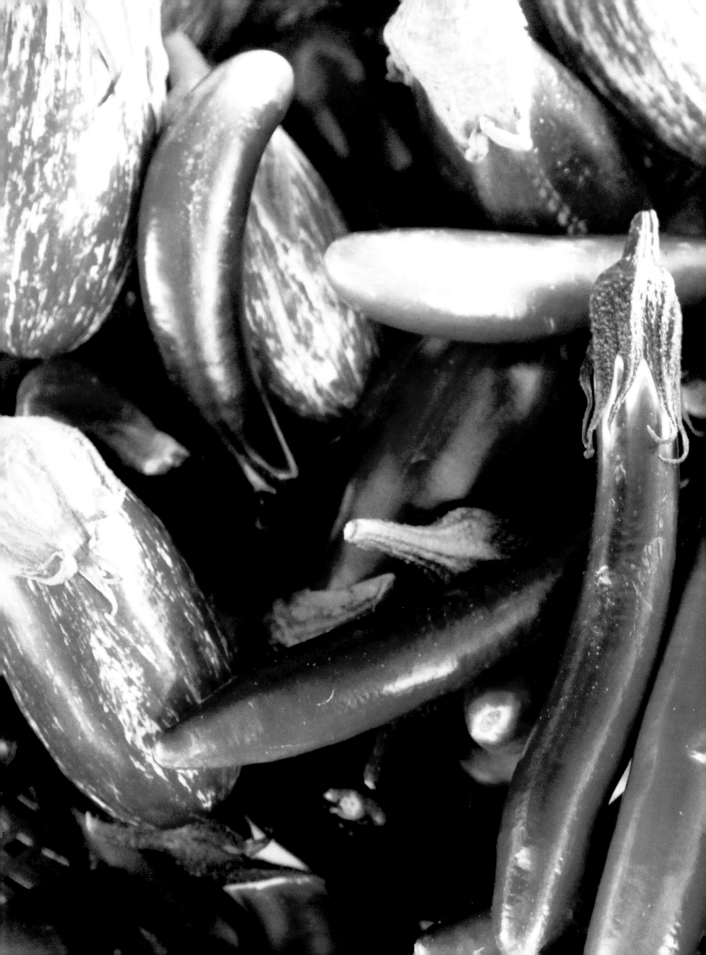

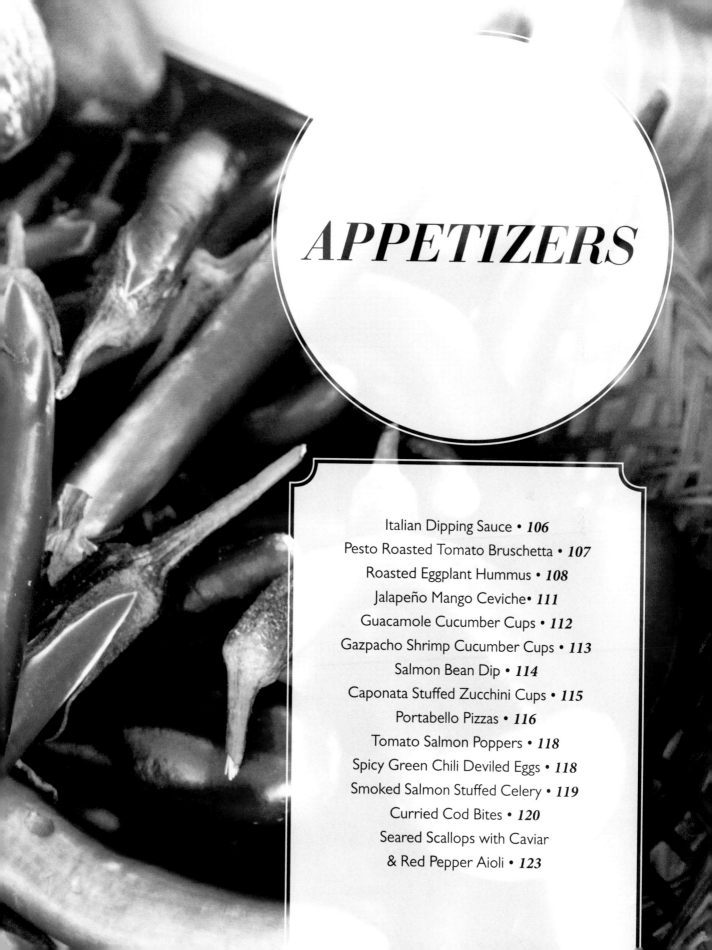

APPETIZERS

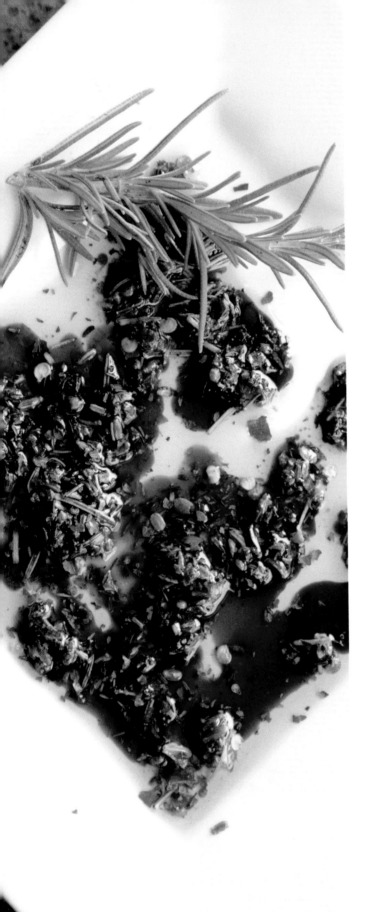

Italian Dipping Sauce

3 Tbsp minced Italian
    flat leaf parsley
2 garlic cloves, finely minced
½ tsp sea salt
⅛-¼ tsp red pepper flakes
½ tsp black pepper
2 tsp fresh oregano
2 tsp fresh rosemary,
    chopped
1 tsp fresh thyme
¼ cup balsamic vinegar
3 Tbsp extra virgin olive oil
1 Tbsp water

2 Tbsp Parmesan or
    Romano cheese,
    finely grated

1. Combine all ingredients except the cheese
and stir.

2. Allow to rest for 30 minutes before enjoying.

3. Add cheese, if using, just before serve.

MAKES ⅔ CUP • SERVES 10

*Fresh and dried herbs both
work well in this recipe.*

Lutein+Zeaxanthin • 70mcg
Omega-3 • 43mg
Vitamin E • 3%DV

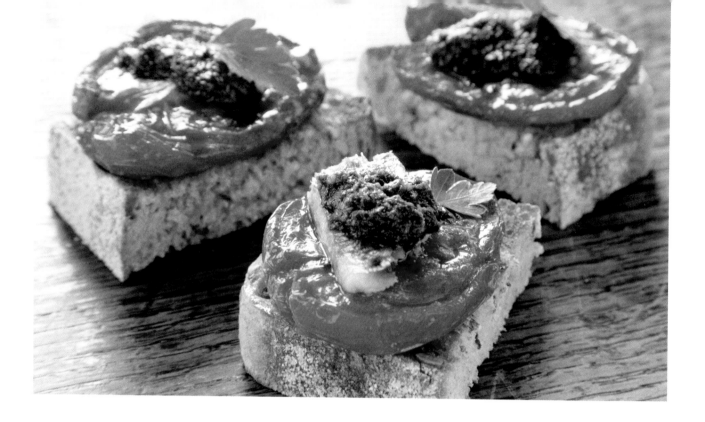

Pesto Roasted Tomato Bruschetta

9 Roma tomatoes, halved lengthwise
¼ tsp sea salt
⅛ tsp black pepper
2 tsp extra virgin olive oil
18 anchovy or sardine fillets
¼ cup Parsley Basil Pesto (page 196)

9 slices whole grain bread, cut in half

Parsley, for garnish

1. Preheat oven to 325°F. Using your fingers, gently squeeze the excess juice from the tomato. In a large glass baking dish, place tomatoes cut side up. Sprinkle with salt and pepper and drizzle with olive oil.

2. Roast tomatoes for 75-90 minutes, or until the base of the tomatoes begin to caramelize. Remove from the oven, place a fillet and a teaspoon of pesto on each tomato, and bake for an additional 5 minutes.

3. Toast the whole grain bread. Cut into wedges slightly larger than tomatoes.

4. Place one pesto roasted tomato on each wedge of bread. Garnish with parsley.

MAKES 18 PIECES • SERVES 9

This appetizer can be enjoy warmed from the oven or served at room temperature.

Lycopene • 2,342mcg
Lutein+Zeaxanthin • 391mcg
Omega-3 • 474mg

Roasted Eggplant Hummus

2 lb eggplant

15 oz can chickpeas, drained and rinsed

¼ cup sun dried tomatoes, drained if packed in oil

2 tsp balsamic vinegar
2 garlic cloves
½ tsp sea salt
¼ tsp black pepper
½ tsp paprika, smoked or sweet
3½ Tbsp extra virgin olive oil
¼ cup marinated artichoke hearts, drained
3 Tbsp Italian flat leaf parsley, minced

1 Tbsp Italian flat leaf parsley, minced
⅛ tsp paprika, smoked or sweet
1½ tsp extra virgin olive oil

1. Preheat oven to 375°F. Cut eggplant in half lengthwise. Sprinkle each half with a pinch of salt. Place eggplant cut-side down on a parchment lined baking sheet. Bake for 30-40 minutes, until halves are soft and flesh is light golden in color. Remove from the oven and allow to cool for 30 minutes.

2. Scoop all the flesh from one of the halves of the eggplant. Create a serving boat from the other half by leaving a ¼" rim of eggplant behind.

3. To a food processor add roasted eggplant, chickpeas, sun dried tomatoes, balsamic vinegar, garlic, salt, pepper, paprika, and olive oil. Puree until smooth in texture.

4. Add artichoke hearts, pulsing until nearly smooth, leaving small pieces behind if desired. Add parsley and briefly pulse to combine.

5. Fill eggplant serving boats with hummus mixture. Drizzle with remaining olive oil and garnish with parsley and paprika.

MAKES 3½ CUPS • SERVES 7

This recipe is great served with crudités, whole grain pita wedges or high-fiber crackers.

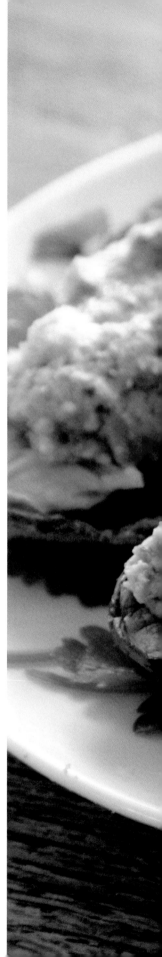

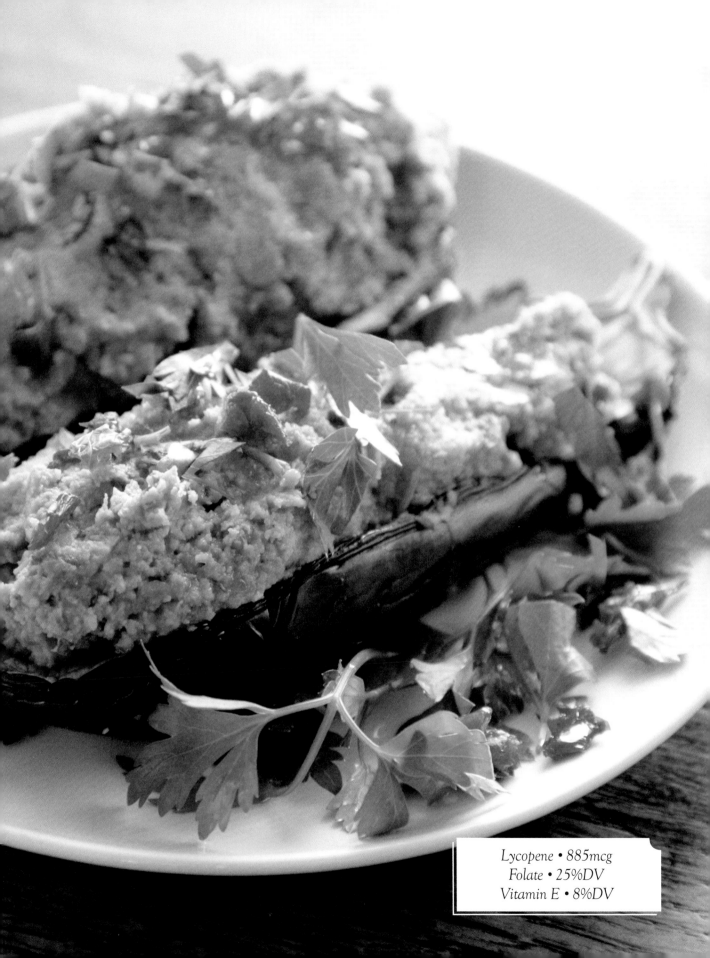

Lycopene • 885mcg
Folate • 25%DV
Vitamin E • 8%DV

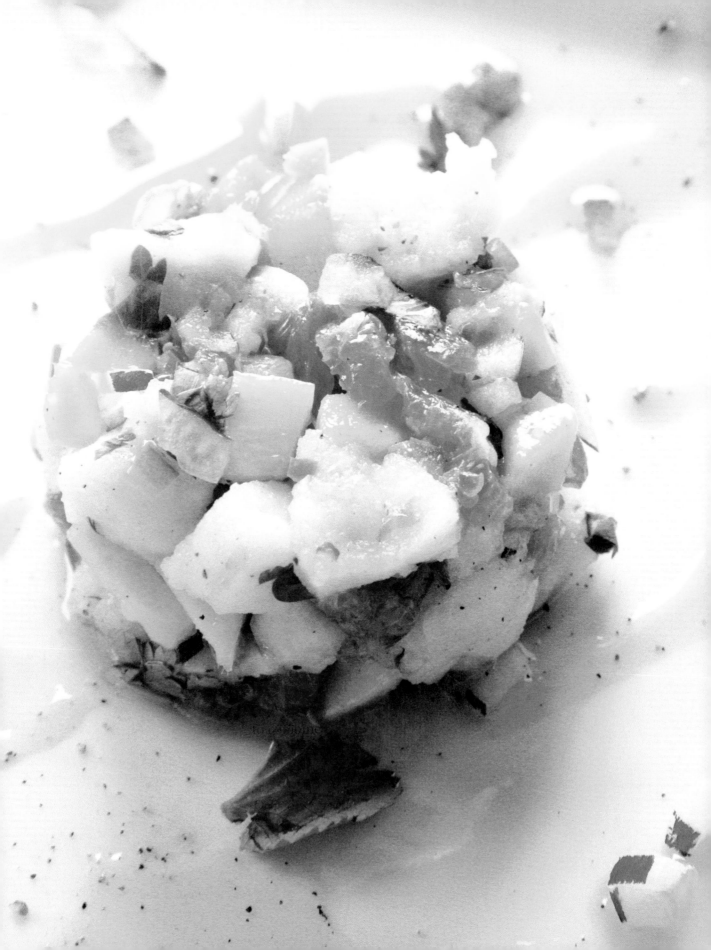

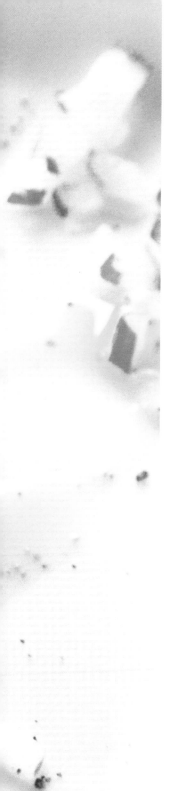

Jalapeño Mango Ceviche

½ lb fresh red snapper,
  ¼" dice
¼ cup lemon juice
¼ cup lime juice

⅓ cup mango, small dice
¼ cup grapefruit, small dice
2 tsp jalapeño, minced, ribs
  and seeds removed
2 Tbsp red onion,
  finely minced
1 Tbsp cilantro, minced
⅛ tsp sea salt
⅛ tsp black pepper

1. Combine snapper, lemon and lime juice in a non-reactive glass or ceramic bowl. The juice should cover the fish completely. Allow to sit refrigerated for 4 hours.

2. Cut a piece of the snapper in half, the fish should look opaque and "cooked". Drain.

3. To a bowl add the snapper, mango, grapefruit, jalapeño, onion and cilantro. Stir to combine.

4. Serve on decoratively garnished plates or in martini glasses.

MAKES 2 CUPS • SERVES 4

Omega-3 • 221mg
Vitamin B12 • 28%DV
Vitamin C • 41%DV

Guacamole Cucumber Cups

2 avocados, ripe

½ cup scallions, sliced
1 Roma tomato, small dice
¼ tsp sea salt
¼ tsp black pepper

½ tsp hot sauce of choice
¼ cup plain Greek yogurt, non- or low-fat
¼ cup cilantro, minced
1 Tbsp lime juice
1 garlic clove, finely minced

2 English cucumbers, cut into 1" slices, peeled if desired

¼ cup cilantro, diced
1 Thai chili or jalapeño, minced

1. In a mixing bowl, mash the avocado with a fork or pastry blender, until smooth or chunky, as desired.

2. Add the next 9 ingredients. Stir to combine.

3. Use a melon baller to create a "cup" for the guacamole by spooning out seeded portion of the cucumber slices, leaving ¼" on the bottom.

4. Spoon 1½ Tbsp guacamole into each cucumber cup. Garnish with cilantro and pepper. Serve immediately or refrigerate until ready to use.

SERVES 8

> Lycopene • 293mcg
> Lutein+Zeaxanthin • 213mcg
> Vitamin C • 16%DV

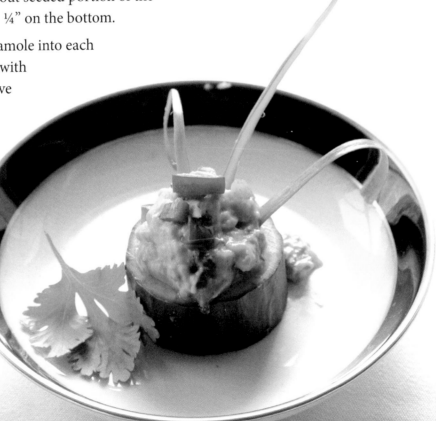

112

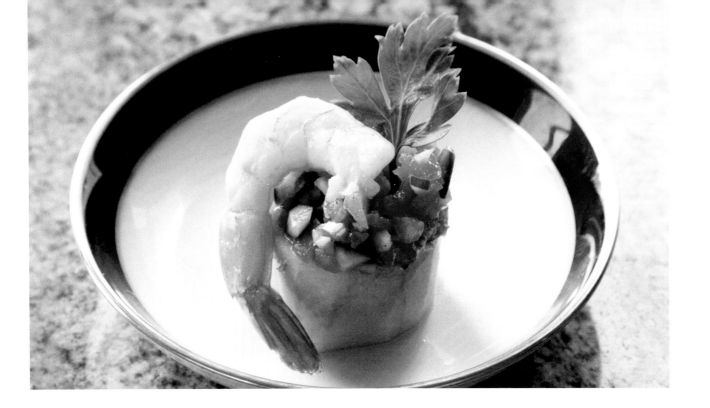

Gazpacho Shrimp Cucumber Cups

½ cup orange bell pepper, roughly chopped
1 cup tomato, diced
⅓ cup onion, roughly chopped
1 garlic clove, minced
½ cup cucumber, roughly diced

1 Tbsp extra virgin olive oil
½-1 jalapeño, ribs and seeds removed, finely minced
½ tsp sea salt
¼ tsp black pepper

2 English cucumbers, cut into 1" slices, peeled, if desired
¾ lb cocktail shrimp, cooked

⅓ cup Italian flat leaf parsley, roughly chopped, for garnish

1. Place bell pepper, tomato, onion, garlic, cucumber, olive oil, jalapeño, salt and pepper into a food processor. Pulse 2-3 times to mince.

2. Use a melon baller to create a "cup" for the gazpacho by spooning out the seeded portion of the cucumber slices, leaving ¼" on the bottom.

3. Spoon 1½ Tbsp of tomato mixture into each cucumber cup. Garnish with shrimp and parsley.

SERVES 10

Omega-3 • 133mg
Vitamin C • 28%DV
Zinc • 5%DV

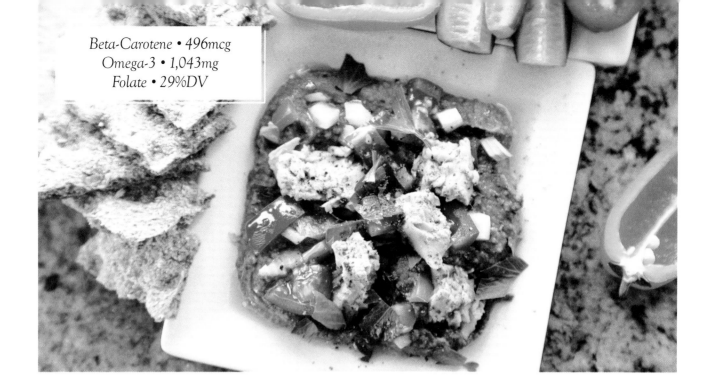

Beta-Carotene • 496mcg
Omega-3 • 1,043mg
Folate • 29%DV

Salmon Bean Dip

1 Tbsp extra virgin olive oil
½ onion, finely diced
1 garlic clove, minced
3 cups black beans,
  drained and rinsed
¼ tsp sea salt
¼ tsp black pepper
⅓ cup plain Greek yogurt,
  non- or low-fat

2 cans (6 oz each) wild
  Alaskan salmon, drained*
½ cup red onion, small dice
1 orange bell pepper,
  small dice
1 jalapeño, ribs and seeds
  removed, diced
1 large tomato, small dice
¼ cup cilantro, minced

¼ cup Italian flat leaf
  parsley, minced
½ tsp extra virgin olive oil
¼ tsp black pepper
¼ tsp paprika,
  smoked or sweet

*12 oz wild salmon poached
and flaked can be substituted
for the canned salmon*

1. For the bean layer, preheat a skillet to medium. Add oil quickly followed by the onions and garlic. Sauté until the onion is softened and translucent, 2-3 minutes.

2. Place cooked onion mixture, beans, salt, pepper and Greek yogurt in a food processor. Puree until smooth. Spread the bean layer on a serving platter.

3. For the salmon layer, arrange the salmon, onion, bell pepper, jalapeño, tomato, parsley and cilantro on top of the bean layer.

4. Drizzle with olive oil, black pepper and paprika, for garnish. Serve with whole grain crackers and vegetables.

SERVES 9

114

Caponata Stuffed Zucchini Cups

4 medium zucchini,
   cut into 1" slices

2 Tbsp extra virgin olive oil
2 shallots, diced
2 garlic cloves, minced
10 sardines,
   drained and mashed
¼ tsp red pepper flakes,
   optional
4 Roma tomatoes, diced
½ medium eggplant,
   peeled and diced
½ tsp paprika,
   smoked or sweet
¼ tsp sea salt
¼ tsp black pepper
½ cup Italian flat leaf parsley,
   chopped

1 tsp extra virgin olive oil
1 Tbsp grated Parmesan
   cheese, grated

1. For the zucchini cups, scoop out inside of the zucchini slices with a melon baller, reserving the portion removed. Leave at least ¼" around the diameter and in the base of the cups to maintain structure during baking. Finely dice the removed portion of the zucchini and set aside.

2. In a large sauté pan over medium heat, add olive oil quickly followed by the shallots, garlic, sardines and red pepper flakes, if using. Sauté for 3 minutes.

3. Add tomato, eggplant, paprika, diced zucchini, salt and pepper. Sauté for 1-2 minutes.

4. Remove from heat, add parsley and stir.

5. Preheat oven to 350°F. Use a pastry brush or clean fingers to lightly coat the zucchini cups with olive oil. Add a heaping portion of the filling to the cups, about 1½ Tbsp each.

6. Place filled cups on a lightly oiled baking sheet. Bake for 20-25 minutes. Remove from oven, top each cup with a pinch of Parmesan cheese, and return to the oven for an additional 3 minutes.

MAKES 20 ZUCCHINI CUPS • SERVES 10

Lutein+Zeaxanthin • 1,897mcg
Omega-3 • 246mg
Vitamin C • 39%DV

Portabello Pizzas

1 tsp dried oregano
1 garlic clove, finely minced
½ tsp dried rosemary,
   chopped
2 Tbsp red onion, diced
Pinch red pepper flakes,
¼ tsp sea salt
¼ tsp black pepper
2 tsp all-purpose flour,
   optional
¾ cup organic tomato puree
8 anchovy fillets,
   finely chopped

6 portabello mushrooms,
   stems and gills removed
1 tsp extra virgin olive oil
1 cup mozzarella cheese,
   grated
4 marinated artichoke
   hearts, cut into wedges
12 kalamata olives,
   pitted and halved
3 Tbsp fresh basil leaves,
   sliced

1. For the pizza sauce combine oregano, garlic, rosemary, onion, red pepper flakes, salt, pepper and flour, if using. Using your hands, rub spices together to bruise. Stir in the tomato puree and anchovy fillets. Set aside.

2. Preheat oven to 400°F. Brush the top of the mushroom caps with olive oil. Place on baking sheet gill side down. Bake for 8-10 minutes. Remove from the oven.

3. Spoon pizza sauce onto each mushroom cap. Decorate with the mozzarella cheese, artichoke hearts and olives.

4. Turn the broiler on to high. Broil until cheese is bubbly and lightly golden.

5. Sprinkle the pizza with the basil to garnish. Cut into quarters and serve immediately.

6-8 APPETIZER PORTIONS •
MAKES 6 PIZZAS

Lycopene • 5,098mcg
Vitamin E • 6%DV
Zinc • 7%DV

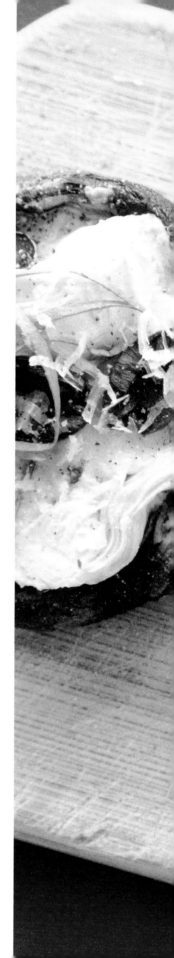

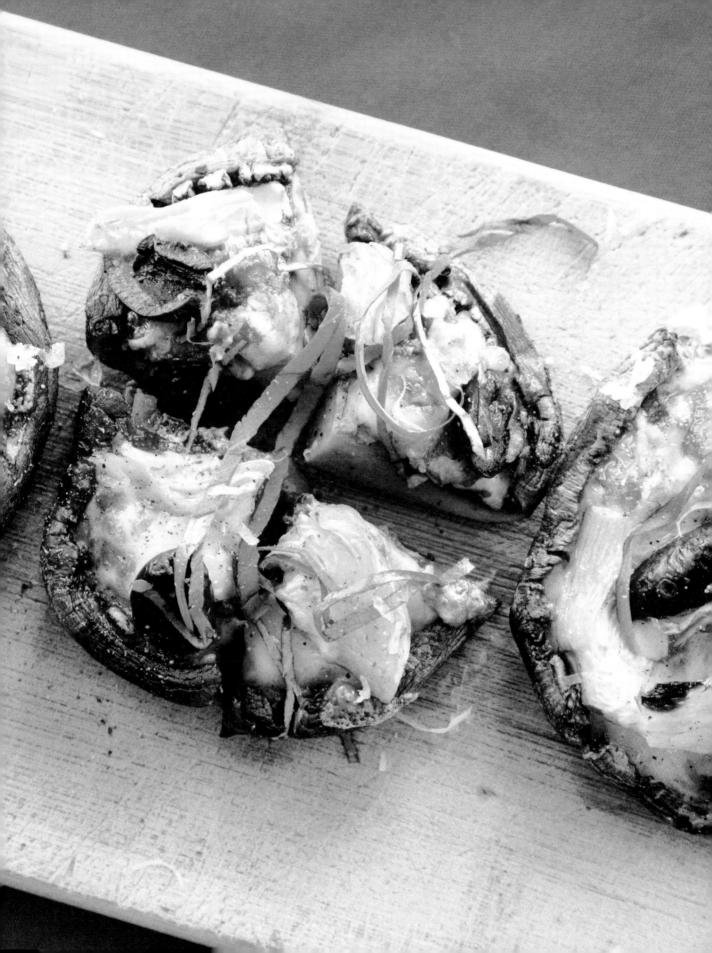

Tomato Salmon Poppers

- 6 oz can wild Alaskan salmon, drained
- ½ cup cooked quinoa, cooled (page 166)
- 3 Tbsp scallions, finely sliced
- 2 Tbsp Italian flat leaf parsley, minced
- 1 Tbsp capers, rinsed if salted, roughly chopped
- 1 garlic clove, finely minced
- ¼ tsp black pepper
- ¼ tsp sea salt
- 1 tsp lemon juice
- 12 small vine-ripened tomatoes
- 1 Tbsp extra virgin olive oil

1. Preheat oven to 375°F. Add to a mixing bowl the first 9 ingredients. Stir to combine. Set aside.

2. Cut a small slice off the top of each tomato. Carefully spoon out the contents of each tomato.

3. Spoon the quinoa-salmon mixture into each of the hollowed tomatoes. Place in an oven safe baking dish. Drizzle lightly with olive oil.

4. Bake for 15-20 minutes, or until heated through and tomatoes start to wilt.

MAKES 12 POPPERS • SERVES 6

Lycopene • 3,191mcg
Lutein+Zeaxanthin • 256mcg
Omega-3 • 748mg

Spicy Green Chili Deviled Eggs

recipe continued on next page ›››

- 6 omega-3 eggs, hard boiled and peeled
- 3 Tbsp Homemade Mayo, (page 178) or store-bought
- 2 tsp anchovy fillets, minced
- ½ tsp turmeric
- ⅛ tsp black pepper
- ¼ tsp hot sauce
- 3 Tbsp canned green chilies, minced
- 2 Tbsp green olives, chopped
- 1 Tbsp cilantro, minced
- 2 Tbsp jalapeño, finely minced
- Sliced olives and paprika, for garnish

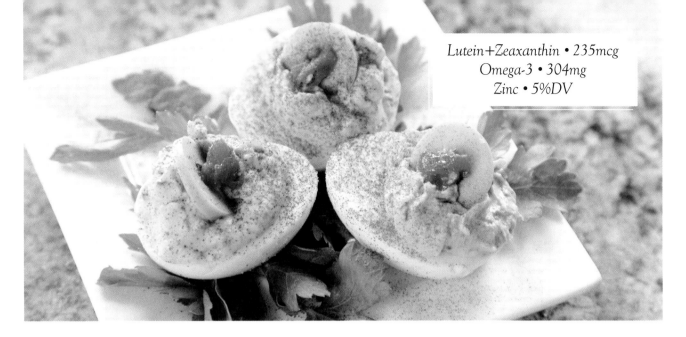

Lutein+Zeaxanthin • 235mcg
Omega-3 • 304mg
Zinc • 5%DV

1. Cut eggs in half. Remove yolks.

2. To a small food processor add the yolks, mayonnaise, anchovies, turmeric, black pepper and hot sauce. Puree until smooth.

3. Add green chilies, olives, cilantro and jalapeño. Pulse once or twice to combine.

4. Spoon the yolk mixture evenly among the halved egg whites.

5. Garnish with sliced olive and paprika. Serve immediately or cover and chill until ready to use.

MAKES 12 HALVES • SERVES 6

Smoked Salmon Stuffed Celery

12.3 oz box tofu, silken firm
1 Tbsp lemon juice
½ tsp lemon zest
2 tsp prepared horseradish
1 Tbsp onion, grated
¼ tsp sea salt
¼ tsp black pepper, to taste

8-10 oz smoked salmon, flaked
1 Tbsp capers, rinsed if salted, roughly chopped
1 Tbsp fresh dill, roughly chopped
8 ribs celery, washed well
½ tsp paprika, sweet or smoked, to garnish

1. Place tofu, lemon juice and zest, horseradish, onion, and salt and pepper into a food processor and process until smooth.

2. Add salmon, capers and dill. Pulse 1-2 times, just to combine.

3. Cut celery into 2" pieces. Spread smoked salmon filling generously. Sprinkle with paprika prior to serving.

MAKES 2⅓ CUPS STUFFING • SERVES 8

Lutein+Zeaxanthin • 130mcg
Omega-3 • 728mg
Vitamin B6 • 15%DV

119

Curried Cod Bites

⅓ cup dry white wine
   or water
⅓ cup light coconut milk
1" knob fresh ginger,
   cut into coins
1 tsp lime zest
¼ tsp turmeric
¼ tsp ground coriander
⅛ tsp ground cumin
¼ tsp sea salt
¼ tsp black pepper

1 Tbsp coconut oil
1½ lb cod, cut into
   24 bite-sized pieces
3 tbsp cilantro, chopped

1. Combine in a sauce pan the wine, coconut milk, ginger, lime zest, turmeric, coriander, cumin, salt and pepper. Bring to a gentle simmer. Simmer for 8-10 minutes.

2. Meanwhile, preheat a non-stick sauté pan to medium high. Add the coconut oil, followed by the cod. Saute 2-3 minutes.

3. Strain the sauce over the cod and simmer 1-2 minutes. Garnish with cilantro. Serve immediately.

MAKES 24 BITES • SERVES 8

Omega-3 • 452mg
Vitamin B12 • 17%DV
Vitamin E • 5%DV

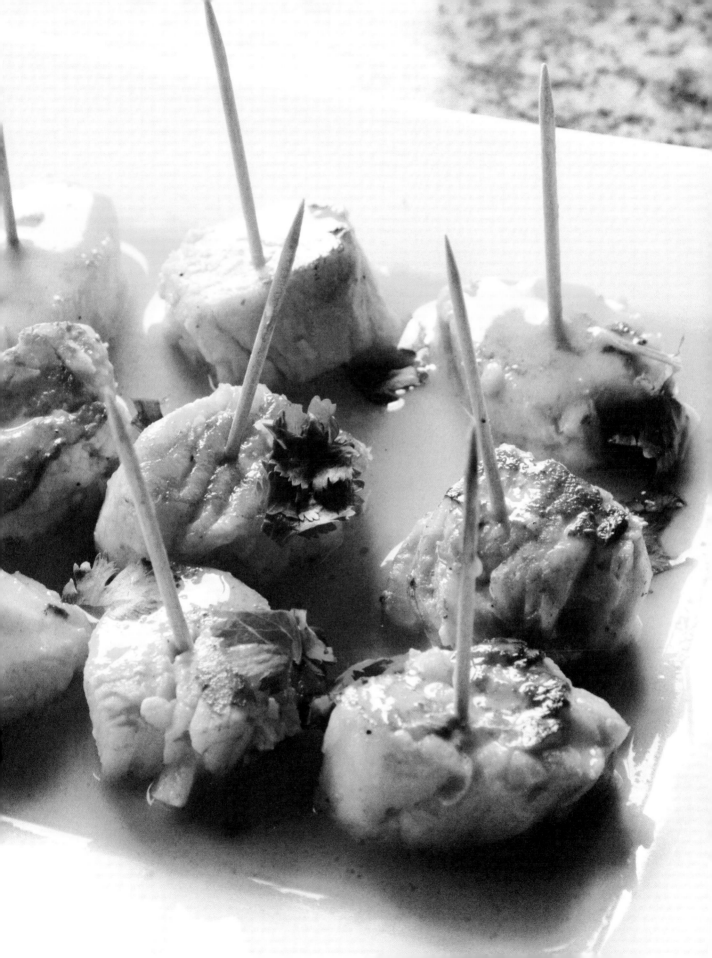

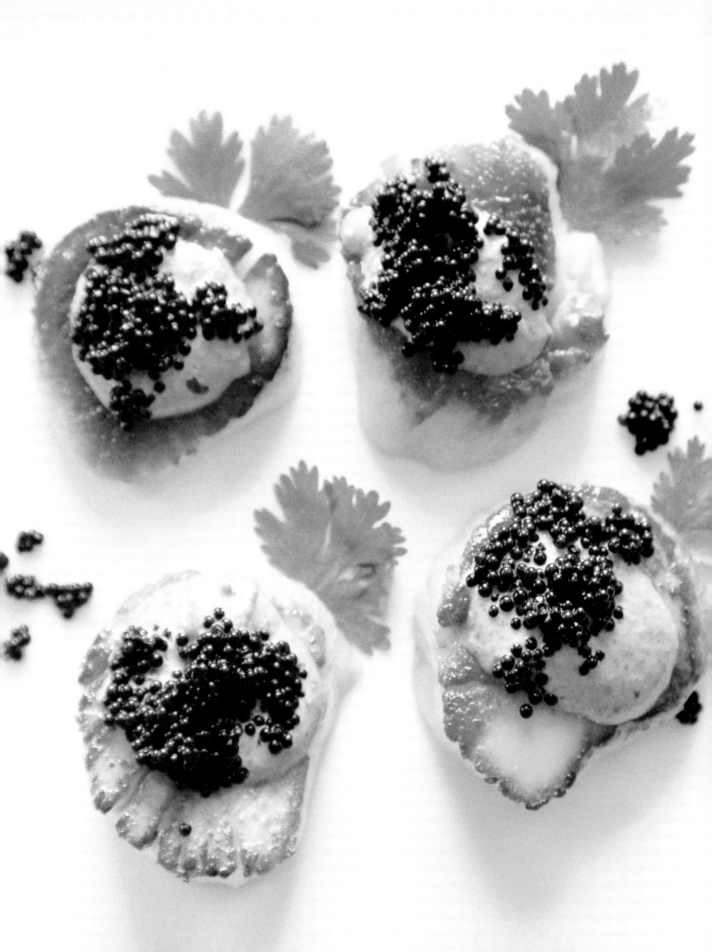

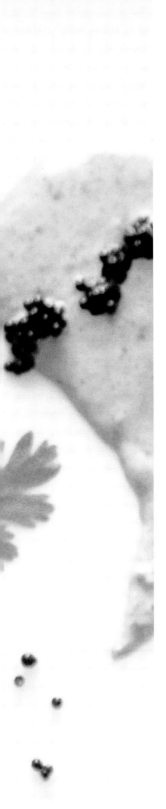

Seared Scallops with Caviar & Red Pepper Aioli

1 Tbsp extra virgin olive oil
12 dry-packed sea scallops
2 Tbsp black caviar
⅔ cup Roasted Red Pepper Aioli (page 179)

¼ cup cilantro, leaves only

1. Preheat a large non-stick sauté pan to medium-high. Add the oil quickly followed by the scallops. Sauté 6-8 minutes until both sides are golden and caramelized, turning only once.

2. Remove from the heat and onto a serving platter.

3. Spoon 2 tsp aioli and ½ tsp caviar onto each scallop. Garnish with cilantro.

SERVES 12

Beta-Carotene • 66mcg
Omega-3 • 353mg
Vitamin B12 • 11%DV

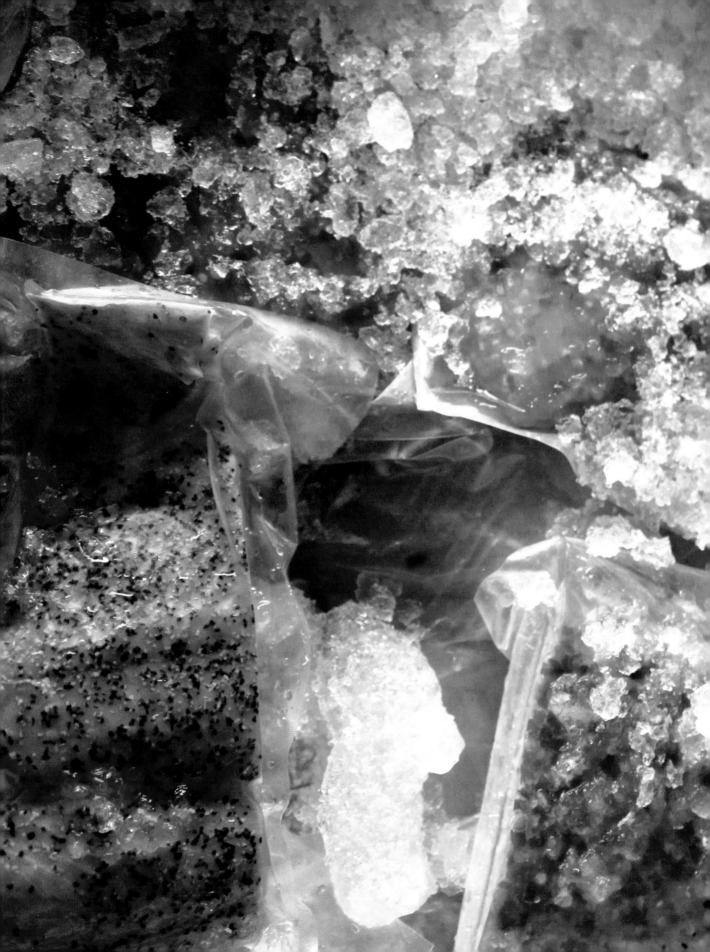

ENTRÉES

Roasted Asian Wild Salmon

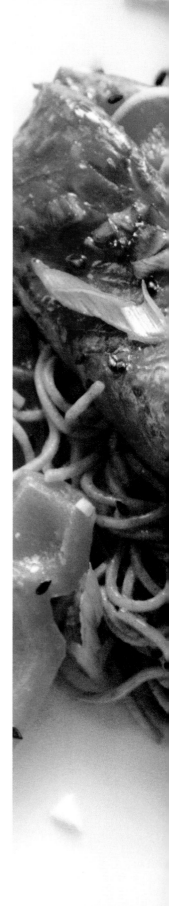

¼ cup Asian dark vinegar or
  rice vinegar
2 garlic cloves, minced
1 Tbsp fresh ginger,
  finely minced
½ tsp wasabi paste
1 tsp dark sesame oil
1 Tbsp extra virgin olive oil
2 Tbsp low-sodium tamari
  or soy sauce

4 wild-caught salmon fillets
  (4-6 oz each), pin-bones
  removed

1 Tbsp extra virgin olive oil
1 red bell pepper, sliced
1 orange bell pepper, sliced

8 oz buckwheat
  soba noodles
2 tsp dark sesame oil
1 Tbsp black sesame seeds

2 Tbsp cilantro
  or parsley, chopped
2 scallions, chopped

1. For the marinade, add the first 7 ingredients to a small bowl and stir to combine.

2. Place the salmon fillets in a small glass dish and cover with half the marinade. Refrigerate for 30 minutes.

3. Preheat oven to 400°F. Place marinated salmon in a lightly greased baking dish and pour the remaining half of the marinade over fillets. Roast for 9-12 minutes, depending on the thickness of the fillet.

4. Preheat a skillet to medium. Add the olive oil quickly followed by the bell peppers. Sauté until crisp tender, 6-8 minutes. Set aside.

5. Bring 3 quarts of water to a rolling boil. Add noodles and stir. Simmer for 6-7 minutes. Drain; toss with sesame oil, black sesame seeds and the reserved bell pepper.

6. Plate soba noodles and vegetables. Top with salmon. Garnish with scallions and cilantro.

SERVES 4

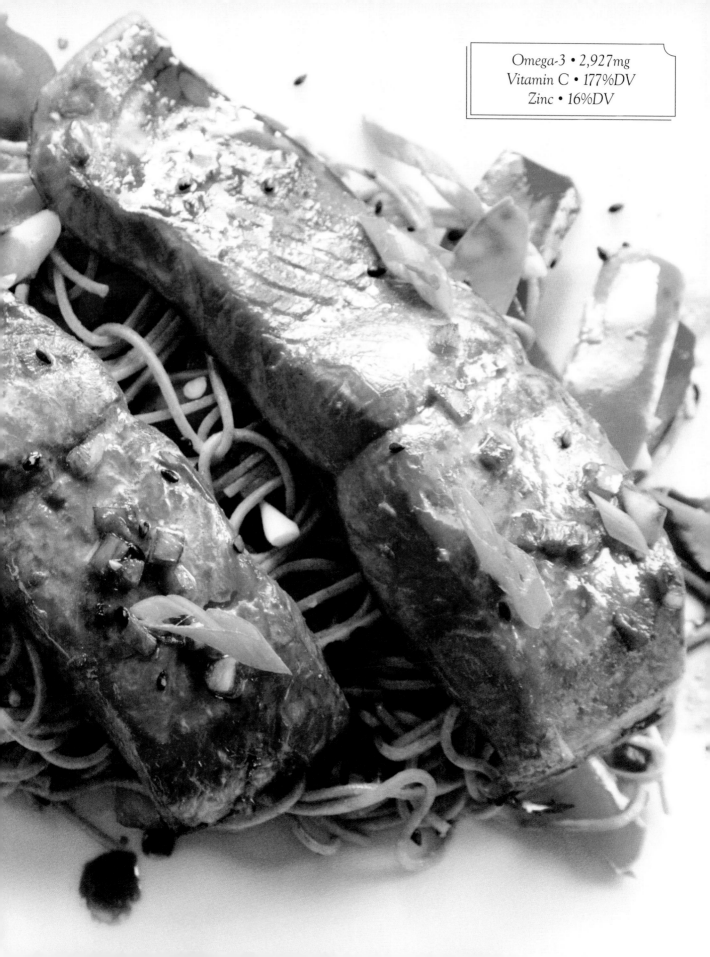

Omega-3 • 2,927mg
Vitamin C • 177%DV
Zinc • 16%DV

Striped Bass with Mediterranean Tapenade

½ cup sun dried tomatoes
½ cup kalamata olives, pitted
14 oz can artichoke hearts, well drained
¼ tsp black pepper
1½ tsp capers, rinsed if salted
1½ Tbsp balsamic vinegar

6 striped bass fillets (6 oz each)
2 Tbsp extra virgin olive oil

3 Tbsp fresh basil, for garnish

1. Preheat oven to 400°F. For the tapenade, roughly chop together the sun dried tomatoes, olives, artichokes hearts, black pepper and capers. Stir in the balsamic vinegar.

2. Place the fillets in an oven safe baking dish. Add equal portions of tapenade to the top of each fillet. Drizzle each fillet with 1 tsp olive oil.

3. Bake in the oven 15-20 minutes. To test for doneness, pierce the thickest part with a fork. The flesh should be opaque and the juices milky-white.

4. Garnish with fresh basil.

SERVES 6

Lycopene • 1,549mcg
Lutein+Zeaxanthin • 292mg
Omega-3 • 1,184mg

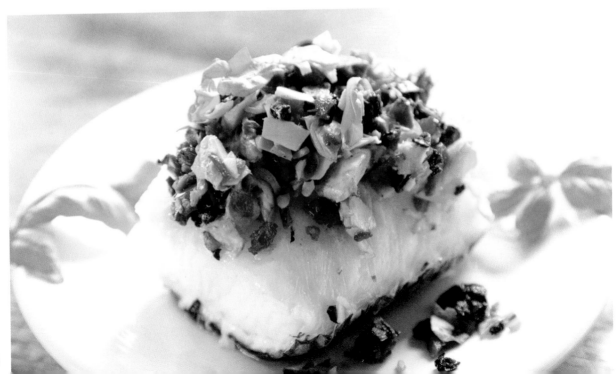

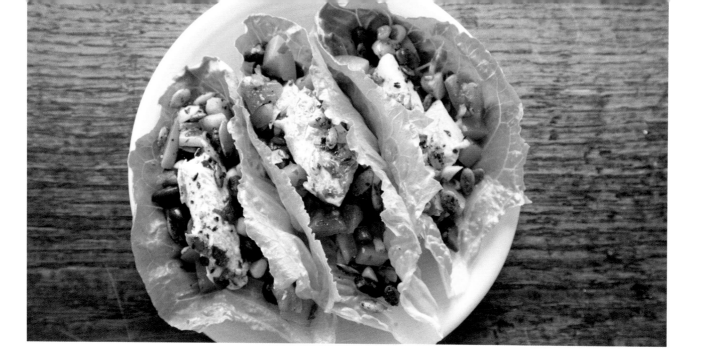

Rainbow Trout Tacos

2 whole rainbow trout
1 Tbsp extra virgin olive oil
Pinch sea salt
Pinch black pepper

15 oz can black beans, drained and rinsed
1 cup frozen corn, thawed
1 orange bell pepper, diced

1 small jalapeño, seeds and ribs removed, finely diced
1 medium tomato, diced
1 small red onion, small dice
¼ cup cilantro, minced
¼ tsp sea salt
¼ tsp black pepper

⅓ cup Achiote Lime Vinaigrette (page 176)
12 romaine lettuce leaves

6 Tbsp Spiced Pepitas roasted with Mexican "Eye Spice" (page 203)
2 limes, cut into 6 wedges for garnish

1. Preheat oven to 400°F. Place the trout in a greased oven safe glass baking dish. Drizzle with olive oil and sprinkle with salt and pepper. Bake for 10-15 minutes, turn over halfway through roasting.

2. In a mixing bowl, combine black beans, corn, bell pepper, jalapeño, tomato, onion, cilantro, salt and pepper. Stir in Achiote Lime Vinaigrette.

3. Debone the trout.

4. To create tacos, place romaine leaves on a platter and divide the black bean and corn mixture between them. Top each with a piece of trout.

5. Garnish with Spiced Pepitas and a wedge of lime.

SERVES 6

Lutein+Zeaxanthin • 1,505mcg
Omega-3 • 1,303mg
Vitamin B12 • 100%DV

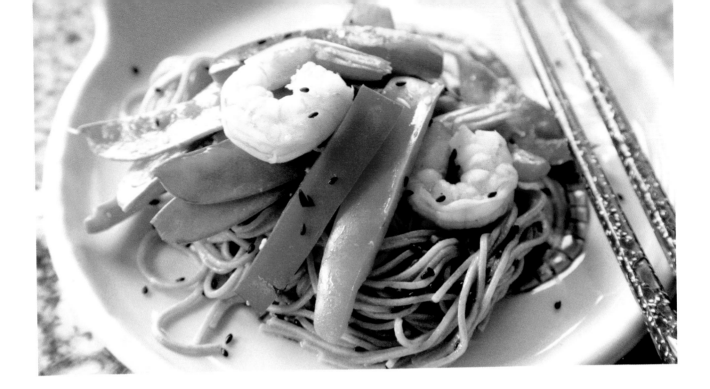

Shrimp, Bell Pepper & Snow Peas

3 quarts boiling water
6 oz buckwheat soba
   noodles
2 tsp sesame oil
1 Tbsp black sesame seeds

1 Tbsp extra virgin olive oil
2 orange bell peppers,
   sliced
1 red bell pepper, sliced
8 oz snow peas,
   strings removed
2 Tbsp filtered water
1¼ lb shrimp,
   peeled and deveined
2 garlic cloves, minced
1 tsp soy sauce or tamari
½ lemon, juiced
½ lemon, cut into wedges

1. Bring water to a rolling boil. Add the noodles and stir. Simmer for 6-7 minutes. Drain and toss with sesame oil and sesame seeds.

2. Preheat a large non-stick sauté pan to medium-high. Add the oil quickly followed by the bell peppers. Stirring constantly, sauté for 1-2 minutes.

3. Add the snow peas and water. Stir, cover and steam for 2 minutes.

4. Uncover and stir in the shrimp, garlic and soy sauce. Sauté an additional 2-3 minutes, stirring until the shrimp are pink.

5. Add the lemon juice and serve with lemon wedges.

SERVES 4

Wild Alaskan salmon may be substituted for the shrimp. Cut 1¼lb of salmon into bite-sized pieces. Add salmon in place of the shrimp. Stir, cover and lower the heat to medium-low. Allow the salmon to cook 3-4 minutes or until cooked through. Add the lemon juice. Serve with lemon wedges.

Lutein+Zeaxanthin • 478mcg
Omega-3 • 691mg
Zinc • 18%DV

Fresh Salmon Burgers

1 lb wild Alaskan salmon
⅔ cup fresh spinach, lightly packed
¼ tsp sea salt
½ tsp black pepper

3 Tbsp onion, finely minced
1 small garlic clove, minced
½ tsp smoked paprika
1 Tbsp extra virgin olive oil

4 whole grain burger buns
4 romaine lettuce leaves
1 large tomato, sliced
½ red onion, sliced

1. For the burgers, place first 7 ingredients into a food processor. Pulse 6-7 times until the salmon has the consistency of ground beef. Shape into 4 patties.

2. Preheat a sauté pan to medium-high. Add half the oil quickly followed by the salmon patties. Sauté 3-4 minutes until lightly golden. Flip burgers over and add remaining olive oil. Sauté an additional 3-4 minutes.

Consider serving with Homemade Mayo (page 178), Roasted Red Pepper Aioli (page 179), or whole grain mustard.

SERVES 4

Lutein+Zeaxanthin • 1,393mcg
Omega-3 • 2,343mg
Vitamin B12 • 59%DV

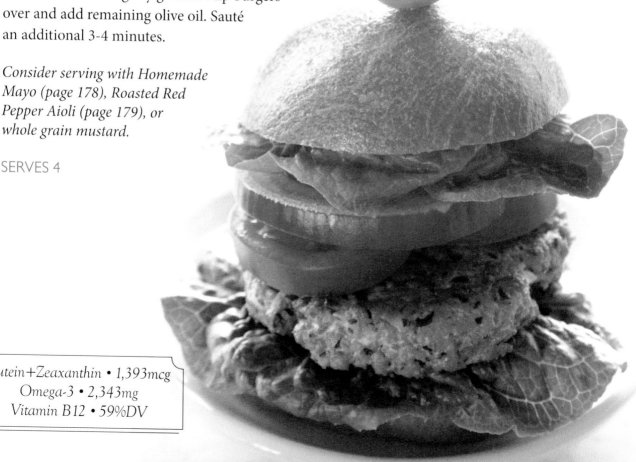

Open-Faced Salmon Pan Bagnat

4 slices whole grain bread
1 garlic clove, peeled

½ cup Sun Dried Tomato Vinaigrette (page 184)
4 slices beefsteak tomato

2 roasted bell peppers, cut into strips (page 179)
4 slices red onion
12 oz lox or smoked salmon, thinly sliced

4 marinated artichoke hearts, cut into wedges
8 kalamata olives, chopped
2 Tbsp Italian flat leaf parsley, chopped
4 basil leaves, torn into small pieces

1. Toast the bread then rub with peeled garlic clove.

2. Place 1 piece of bread on each serving plate. Drizzle the bread with 1 Tbsp vinaigrette.

3. Place tomato, bell pepper and onions on top of bread. Next, add the lox. Garnish with artichokes, olives, parsley and basil.

4. Drizzle each sandwich with 1 Tbsp vinaigrette.

SERVES 4   *Eat with a knife and fork!*

Lycopene • 2,600mcg
Lutein+Zeaxanthin • 456mcg
Omega-3 • 1,767mg

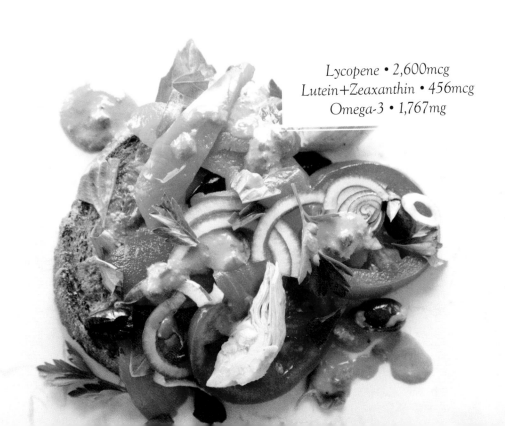

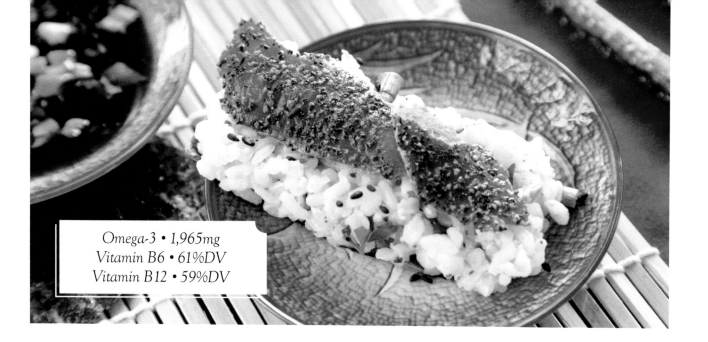

Omega-3 • 1,965mg
Vitamin B6 • 61%DV
Vitamin B12 • 59%DV

Easy Smoked Salmon Sushi

2 Tbsp Asian dark vinegar
2 garlic cloves, minced
2 tsp ginger, finely minced
½-1 tsp wasabi paste
1 tsp dark sesame oil
1 Tbsp extra virgin olive oil
2 Tbsp soy sauce or tamari
3 Tbsp rice wine or water

1 cup short grain
   brown rice, uncooked
1¾ cup water or stock
¼ tsp sea salt
2 Tbsp rice vinegar
½ cup parsley, minced
½ cup scallions, sliced

30 nori sheets,
    snack-size (1.5"×3.5")
1 lb smoked salmon
   or lox
   or sushi grade salmon,
   thinly sliced

Small bowl of water for
   dipping fingers
Waxed paper

1. For the sauce combine the first 8 ingredients and set aside.

2. For the rice, combine rice, water and salt in heavy pot. Bring rice to a simmer over medium heat. Turn heat to low, stir and cover. Allow to cook for 45 minutes. Remove from the heat with the lid still on, allowing rice to steam for another 10 minutes.

3. Turn the rice out onto a cookie sheet and sprinkle with vinegar, parsley and scallions. Lightly mix.

4. To assemble, lay out half the nori sheets. Dip fingers in water then take a portion of the rice and mound on top of each nori sheet. Lay a piece of salmon on top of the rice.

5. Refrigerate or serve immediately with the sauce and extra nori.

MAKES 12-15 PIECES • SERVES 4

133

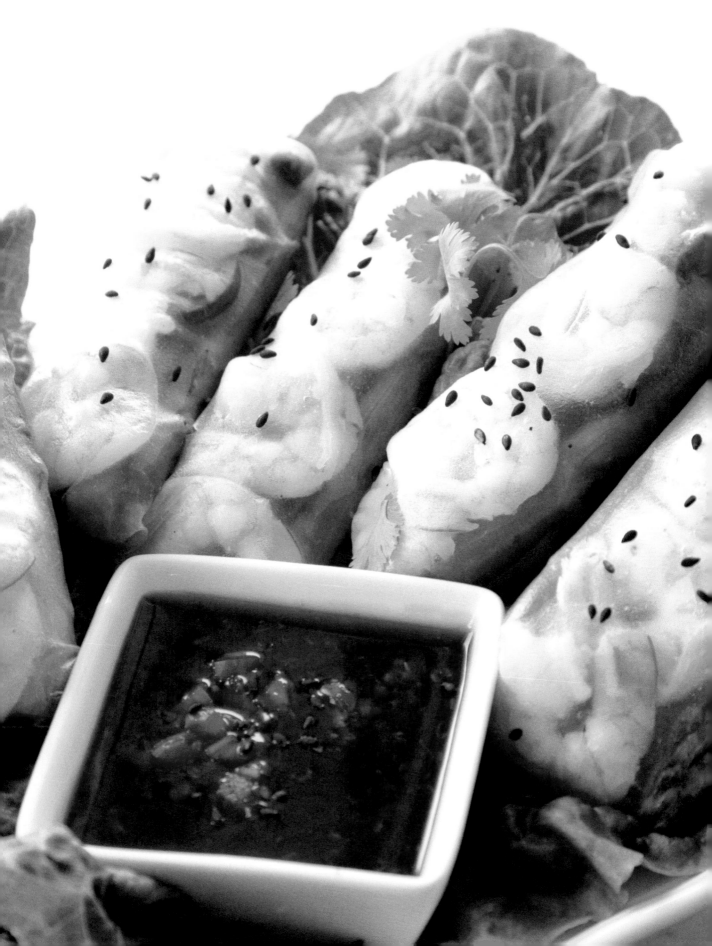

Shrimp & Sweet Potato Spring Rolls

1 small sweet potato, julienned (1¼lb)
1 lb asparagus
1 lb shiitake or crimini mushroom caps
1 Tbsp extra virgin olive oil
⅛ tsp sea salt

2 garlic cloves, finely minced
2 tsp fresh ginger, grated
1 tsp wasabi
4 tsp rice vinegar
2 Tbsp soy sauce or tamari
⅓ cup filtered water
1 tsp arrowroot starch
2 Tbsp fresh cilantro or mint, minced
1 Tbsp Thai basil, minced, optional
½ tsp red pepper flakes

¾ lb cooked shrimp, peeled and deveined

16 romaine lettuce leaves
16 rice paper rounds

1. Preheat oven to 375°F. Place sweet potato on a baking sheet. Place asparagus and mushrooms on a separate baking sheet. Drizzle each baking sheet with olive oil and sprinkle with the sea salt.

2. Lightly roast the asparagus and mushrooms for 13-18 minutes; lightly roast the sweet potato 20-25 minutes, stirring each once or twice.

3. For the dipping sauce, combine in a small microwaveable bowl the garlic, ginger, wasabi, rice vinegar, soy sauce and water. Stir in the arrowroot starch until dissolved. Microwave the mixture to lightly thicken, stirring every 30 seconds.

4. Remove from the microwave and add the basil, cilantro and red pepper flakes.

5. Place romaine leaves on a serving platter. Set aside.

6. To create the spring rolls, dip 1 rice paper round in room temperature water. Lay on a flat surface. Decorate with shrimp, asparagus, mushrooms and sweet potatoes. Fold the top and the bottom portions of the rice paper over the vegetables. Fold the sides in to seal.

7. Enjoy each spring roll wrapped in one leaf of romaine lettuce and dipped in the dipping sauce.

Lutein+Zeaxanthin • 3,536mcg
Omega-3 • 471mg
Folate • 59%DV

MAKES 16 ROLLS • SERVES 4

Carrots & Kale Couscous with Salmon

1 Tbsp extra virgin olive oil
2 garlic cloves, minced
2 small carrots, diced
2 cups kale, stems removed, roughly chopped
1 Tbsp filtered water
1¼ cups stock of choice or water
½ tsp sea salt
¼ tsp black pepper
1 cup whole grain couscous, uncooked

6 salmon fillets (6 oz each), with skin
Pinch sea salt & black pepper
1 Tbsp extra virgin olive oil
¼ cup dry white wine or water

Parsley, roughly chopped & paprika, sweet or smoked, for garnish

1. Preheat a 2½ qt sauce pan to medium high. Add the olive oil quickly followed by the garlic, carrots and kale. Sauté 2-3 minutes.

2. Add 1 Tbsp water and cover. Cook 3-4 additional minutes, until carrots are crisp tender. Add the stock or water, salt and pepper. Bring to a simmer.

3. Stir in the couscous. Cover and remove from the heat. Allow to rest 5-10 minutes.

4. Sprinkle the salmon with a pinch of salt and pepper. Preheat a large lidded skillet to medium. Add the olive oil quickly followed by the salmon, skin side down. Sauté 1 minute.

5. Add the white wine or water. Cover and cook 6-8 minutes or until salmon is cooked through.

6. To serve, fluff the couscous with a fork. Spoon onto a serving platter. Place the salmon fillet on top. Garnish with parsley and paprika.

SERVES 6

Lutein+Zeaxanthin • 8,929mcg
Omega-3 • 3,473mg
Vitamin B12 • 89%DV

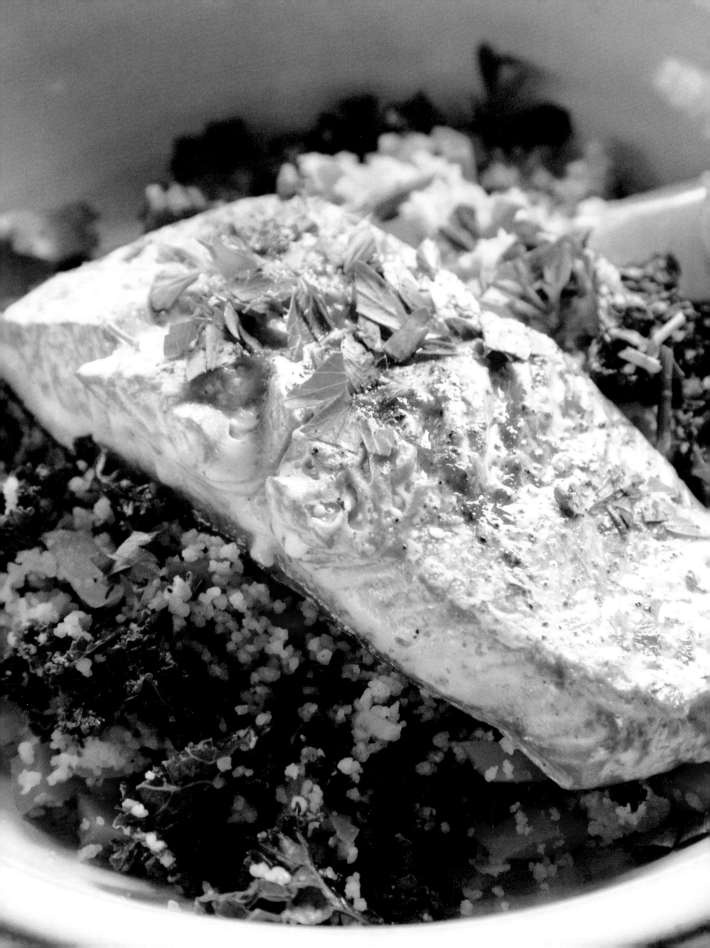

Tilapia with California Chili Mole

1 Tbsp extra virgin olive oil
6 tilapia fillets
1 cup California Chili Mole (page 177)

1 Tbsp extra virgin olive oil
1 large garlic clove, minced
16 oz fresh spinach
2 Tbsp filtered water
¼ tsp sea salt
¼ tsp black pepper
¼ cup cilantro, roughly chopped

1. Preheat oven to 400°F. Place the tilapia fillets in a lightly oiled glass baking dish. Top each fillet with 2 Tbsp of the mole. Bake 9-12 minutes, until flaky.

2. For the spinach, preheat a very large sauté pan up to medium. Add the olive oil and garlic. Stir for 10 seconds. Add the spinach and water. Stir and cover to wilt the spinach.

3. Remove from the heat and drain. Sprinkle with salt and pepper.

4. Garnish with fresh cilantro. Serve with the extra warmed California Chili Mole.

SERVES 6

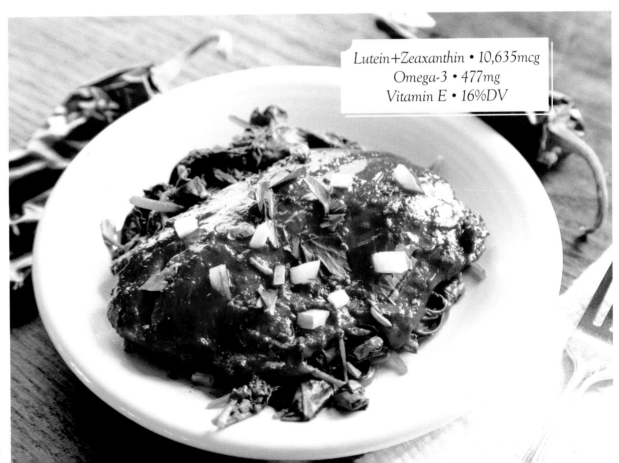

Lutein+Zeaxanthin • 10,635mcg
Omega-3 • 477mg
Vitamin E • 16%DV

Shiitake Sesame Salmon & Veggies

8 oz brown rice noodles
1 tsp dark sesame oil

2 tsp extra virgin olive oil
2 garlic cloves, minced
1 Tbsp fresh ginger, grated
1 cup carrots, julienned
2 cups broccoli florets
8 oz snow peas
1 cup shiitake or crimini mushrooms, sliced
2 Tbsp filtered water

½ cup dried shiitake mushrooms
2 Tbsp sesame seeds
⅛ tsp garlic powder
¼ tsp sea salt
¼ tsp black pepper
2 Tbsp extra virgin olive oil
1½ lb wild Alaskan salmon, cut into 6 equal portions
⅓ cup water

¼ cup scallions, sliced
¼ cup cilantro, roughly chopped

1. Cook the noodles according to package directions. Add sesame oil and set aside.

2. For the vegetables, preheat a large skillet to medium high. Add olive oil quickly followed by the garlic, ginger, carrots and broccoli. Sauté for 2 minutes.

3. Reduce heat to medium-low, add snow peas, mushrooms and 2 Tbsp water. Cover and let steam for 3 minutes until vegetables are crisp tender.

4. Toss the vegetables with the noodles.

5. To prepare the salmon coating, place the shiitake mushrooms in a food processor and pulse to create a coarse powder. Add sesame seeds, garlic powder, salt and pepper. Pulse once to combine.

6. Place coating on a flat platter. Dredge the salmon fillets to coat all sides.

7. Preheat a large covered skillet to medium high. Add the oil and salmon, skin side up. Sauté for 2 minutes. Turn the fillets over.

8. Add water and cover the skillet. Turn the heat down to low. Steam for 7-9 minutes or until fillets are cooked through.

9. To serve, place noodles, vegetables and salmon on a platter and garnish with scallions and cilantro.

SERVES 6

Lutein+Zeaxanthin • 807mcg
Omega-3 • 2,343mg
Zinc • 15%DV

Turmeric Chicken

1 tsp turmeric
1 tsp ground cardamom
1 tsp ground coriander
1 tsp powdered ginger
1 tsp garlic powder
1 tsp cinnamon
¼ tsp sea salt
½ tsp black pepper
1 Tbsp lemon juice
1 Tbsp extra virgin olive oil

2 Tbsp extra virgin olive oil, divided
1¼ lb boneless skinless chicken breasts, sliced or pounded thinly
1 small red onion, small dice
1 orange bell pepper, diced
2 cups broccoli florets, bite-sized pieces
½ cup stock or water
¼ cup plain Greek yogurt, non- or low-fat
¼ cup Italian flat leaf parsley, minced

1. For the marinade, combine turmeric, cardamom, coriander, ginger, garlic, cinnamon, salt and pepper. Stir to combine. Add the lemon juice and olive oil. Stir again.

2. Pour the marinade over the chicken in a glass bowl. Rub the marinade into the chicken. Cover and refrigerate 30 minutes or until ready to cook.

3. Preheat a large nonstick skillet to medium high. Add 1 tbsp olive oil quickly followed by the chicken. Lightly brown chicken on both sides until cooked through. Remove the chicken, set aside and cover to keep warm.

4. Add the onions, bell pepper, broccoli and the reserved olive oil, if necessary. Sauté 8-10 minutes, stirring frequently until vegetables are crisp tender.

5. Reduce the heat to medium-low, add the stock or water and the yogurt.

6. Stir and simmer for 1 minute. Serve with the chicken. Garnish with parsley.

SERVES 4

Vitamin B6 • 51%DV
Vitamin C • 171%DV
Vitamin E • 14%DV

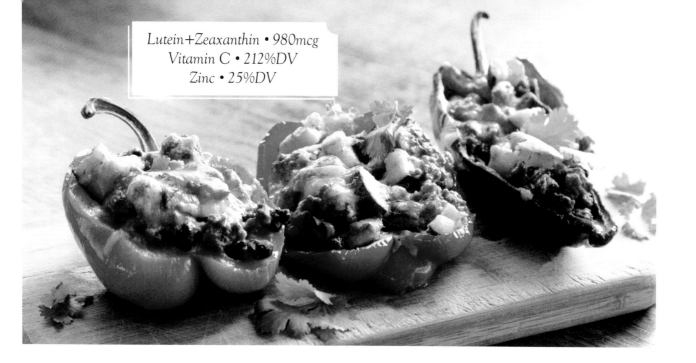

Lutein+Zeaxanthin • 980mcg
Vitamin C • 212%DV
Zinc • 25%DV

Stuffed Peppers

4 poblano chili peppers, halved lengthwise

2 bell peppers, halved lengthwise

1½ Tbsp extra virgin olive oil, divided

1 lb grass-fed ground bison or beef

1 medium red onion, small dice

2 garlic cloves, minced

14.5 oz can diced tomatoes

2 cups zucchini, ½" dice

1 cup black beans, drained and rinsed

2 tsp mild chili powder

¼ tsp ground cumin

¼ tsp sea salt

¼ tsp black pepper

½ cup organic cheddar cheese, grated

1. Preheat oven to 375°F. Remove the ribs and seeds from the halved poblano and bell peppers. Lightly rub the peppers with ½ Tbsp olive oil.

2. Place on a baking sheet cut-side down and roast for 15-18 minutes. Remove from the oven.

3. While the peppers are roasting, preheat a large sauté pan over medium high. Add the remaining oil quickly followed by the bison, onion, garlic, and a pinch of salt. Sauté until the onions are soft and the bison is lightly brown and fully cooked, about 8-10 minutes total.

4. Add the tomatoes, zucchini, black beans, chili powder, cumin, salt and pepper. Sauté 3-4 minutes.

5. Remove from the heat and spoon into the peppers. Place the stuffed peppers back into a baking dish. Pour any accumulated liquid over the top.

6. Sprinkle with cheese. Bake uncovered for 15 minutes until cheese is lightly golden.

SERVES 8

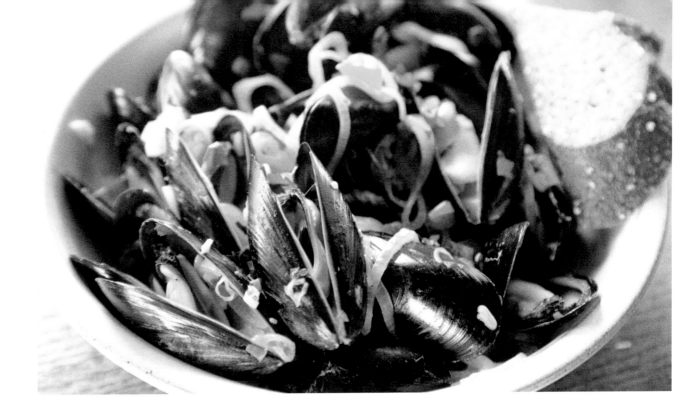

Saffron, Thyme & Shallot Mussels

1 ½ cups high-quality stock, chicken or vegetable
Pinch of saffron

1 Tbsp extra virgin olive oil or grass-fed butter
2 shallots, thinly sliced

2 garlic clove, minced
1 orange bell pepper, small dice
½ tsp fresh thyme, leaves only
Pinch red pepper flakes
¼ tsp sea salt

¼ tsp black pepper
4 lb live mussels, cleaned and debearded

⅓ cup Italian flat leaf parsley

1. Heat the stock to steaming hot on the stovetop or in the microwave. Remove from the heat and add the saffron. Set aside.

2. Preheat lidded Dutch oven to medium high. Add oil quickly followed by the shallots, garlic and bell pepper. Sauté until they begin to soften, 1-2 minutes.

3. Add the infused stock, thyme, red pepper flakes, salt and pepper. Allow to simmer 1 additional minute.

4. Add the mussels, stir and cover. Cook for 5-9 minutes, until the mussels have opened.

5. Garnish with parsley and serve.

12 APPETIZER PORTIONS

Omega-3 • 734mg
Vitamin B12 • 299%DV
Zinc • 17%DV

Coconut, Garlic & Ginger Mussels

1 Tbsp coconut oil
or grass-fed butter
1 Tbsp fresh ginger, grated
2 garlic cloves, minced
2 shallots, diced
1 orange bell pepper,
small dice

½ tsp turmeric
¼ tsp sea salt
¼ tsp black pepper
1 Thai chili, diced
¾ cup vegetable stock
¾ cup light coconut milk

4 lb live mussels, cleaned
and debearded

⅓ cup cilantro, roughly
chopped

1. Preheat a lidded Dutch oven to medium high. Add coconut oil quickly followed by the ginger, garlic, shallots and bell pepper. Sauté until softened, 1-2 minutes.

2. Add the turmeric, salt, pepper, Thai chili, stock and coconut milk. Simmer for 2-3 minutes on medium-low.

3. Add the mussels, stir and cover. Cook for 5-9 minutes, until mussels have opened.

4. Garnish with cilantro and serve.

12 APPETIZER PORTIONS

This recipe is delicious served with crusty sprouted whole grain bread.

Omega-3 • 727mg
Vitamin B12 • 299%DV
Vitamin C • 53%DV

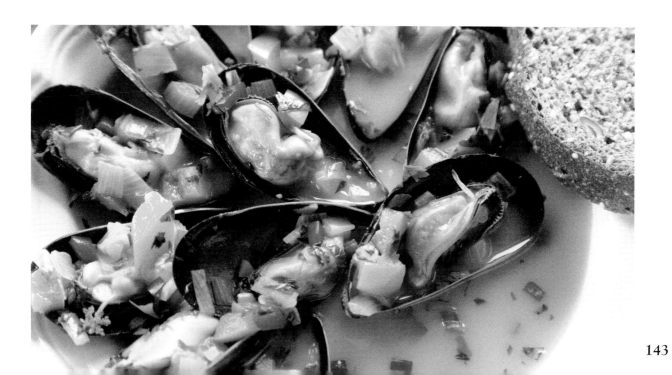

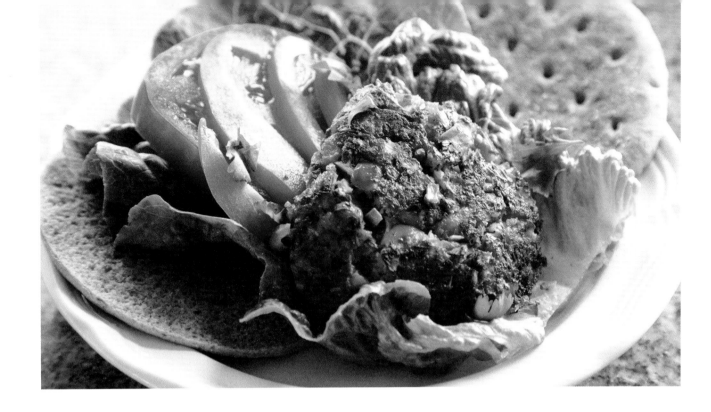

Veggie Burgers

½ cup red onion,
roughly chopped

1 cup asparagus,
coarsely chopped

1 cup orange pepper,
roughly chopped

2 garlic cloves, minced

⅓ cup parsley, lightly packed

½ tsp sea salt

½ tsp black pepper

2 tsp balsamic vinegar

¼ cup ground flax seed

1 omega-3 egg

3 slices hearty whole grain
bread, torn into pieces
(1¾ cup lightly packed)

2 Tbsp extra virgin olive oil

1. Add all the ingredients except the olive oil to a food processor. Pulse 4-5 times, until vegetables are small pea size.

2. Allow to rest 15 minutes.

3. Form into 6 patties.

4. Preheat a non-stick sauté pan to medium-low. Add 1 Tbsp olive oil and the veggie burgers. Sauté 8-10 minutes, until golden. Turn over. Add an additional Tbsp olive oil. Sauté until golden, another 6-8 minutes.

SERVES 4

Consider serving with Tzatziki Dip (page 192).

Lutein+Zeaxanthin • 646mcg
Omega-3 • 1,772mg
Vitamin C • 97%DV

Curried Vegetables & Tofu

1 Tbsp extra virgin olive oil
½ tsp mustard seeds
1 Tbsp ground coriander
2 garlic cloves, minced
2 tsp fresh ginger, grated
½ onion, diced
¾ tsp turmeric
½ tsp sea salt

¼ tsp black pepper

1 cup carrots, diced
1 orange bell pepper,
 1" dice
½ lb Brussels sprouts, halved

1 Thai red chili
 or Serrano pepper,
 finely minced, optional
7 oz firm tofu, ½" cubes
½ cup light coconut milk
¼ cup filtered water

1. Preheat a large covered pot to medium. Add olive oil quickly followed by the mustard seeds, coriander, ginger and garlic. Sauté briefly. Add the onion, turmeric, salt and pepper. Sauté 2-3 minutes until the onion begins to soften.

2. Stir in the carrot, bell pepper, Brussels sprouts and chili, if using. Sauté for another 2-3 minutes.

3. Add the tofu, coconut milk and water. Cover and simmer over low heat for an additional 10-15 minutes until vegetables are crisp tender, stirring once or twice.

MAKES 5 CUPS

Consider serving with 2 cups cooked brown rice.

Beta-Carotene • 3,586mcg
Lutein+Zeaxanthin • 1,013mcg
Vitamin C • 177%DV

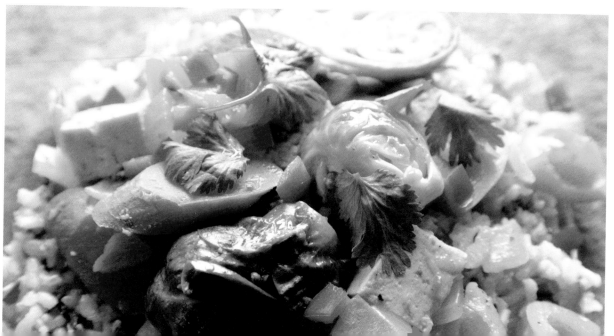

Coconut Turkey Tenders

1 recipe Indian Yogurt
  Marinade (page 192),
  divided

½ tsp turmeric
1 tsp paprika,
  sweet or smoked
⅛ tsp onion powder
½ tsp sea salt
¼ tsp black pepper
1 tsp arrowroot starch
1 lb turkey breast, cut into
  3" strips, patted dry with
  a paper towel

1 cup unsweetened
  shredded coconut
2 Tbsp extra virgin olive oil

1. Preheat oven to 400°F. Place one half of the Indian Yogurt Marinade in a serving bowl. Reserve the other half in a mixing bowl.

2. Combine the turmeric, paprika, onion powder, salt, pepper, and arrowroot starch. Add the turkey strips and stir to coat.

3. Place the shredded coconut onto a plate. Dip the turkey strips into the reserved yogurt marinade and then into the shredded coconut. Place on a parchment lined baking sheet. Wash hands thoroughly. Drizzle oil over the top.

4. Bake 18-22 minutes, until turkey is cooked through and coconut is lightly browned.

5. Serve with veggies for the kids, young and old, to dip into the yogurt sauce.

SERVES 4 ADULTS
OR 6-8 CHILDREN

Beta-Carotene • 212mcg
Vitamin B6 • 43%DV
Zinc • 18%DV

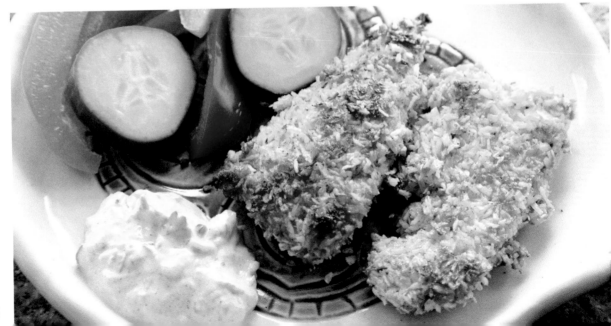

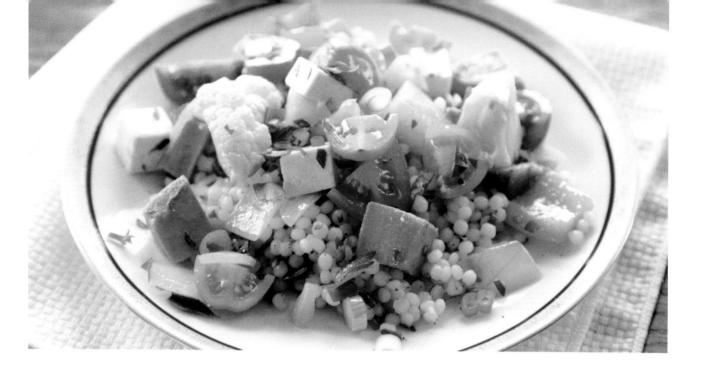

Roasted Vegetables & Israeli Couscous

1 ½ cups Israeli couscous,
      uncooked
   2 tsp extra virgin olive oil
1 ¾ cups water
   ½ tsp sea salt

   ½ medium onion, ½" dice

   2 cups sweet potatoes, ½"
      dice
   2 cups cauliflower,
      cut into bite-sized florets
   ½ orange bell pepper, diced
   8 oz extra firm tofu, ½"
      cubes
   1 Tbsp balsamic vinegar

   1 Tbsp extra virgin olive oil
   ¼ tsp sea salt
   ¼ tsp black pepper
   ¼ cup parsley,
      roughly chopped
   ¼ cup scallions,
      roughly chopped
   ½ cup cherry tomatoes,
      halved

1. For the couscous, preheat a 2½ quart sauce pan to medium. Add olive oil quickly followed by the couscous. Saute 2 minutes, stirring occasionally.

2. Add water and salt. Bring to a simmer and cover. Simmer for 8-10 minutes.

3. To roast the vegetables, preheat oven to 375°F. In a large bowl, combine onion, sweet potato, cauliflower, bell pepper, tofu, balsamic vinegar, olive oil, salt and pepper. Stir to evenly coat.

4. Pour onto a lightly greased baking sheet. Bake for 30-40 minutes, stirring twice.

5. Stir parsley and scallions into the couscous. Serve with roasted vegetables .

6. Garnish with cherry tomatoes.

MAKES 9 CUPS • 6 SERVINGS

Lycopene • 320mcg
Lutein+Zeaxanthin • 227mcg
Vitamin C • 97%DV

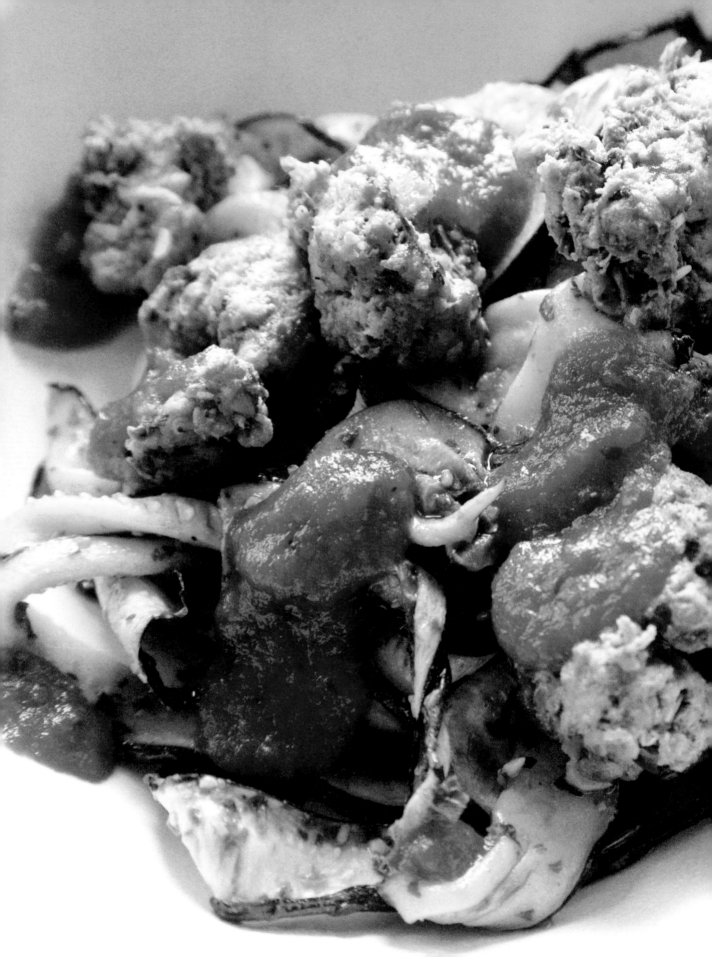

Italian Sausage & Fresh Pesto Pappardelle

½ recipe Fresh Marinara
(page 195)

2 garlic cloves, minced
1 tsp oregano, rubbed
2 tsp Italian herb mix
1 tsp fennel
1 tsp rosemary
1 tsp paprika,
smoked or sweet
¼ tsp black pepper
¼ tsp red pepper flakes,
¾ tsp sea salt
1 lb ground turkey,
93% lean
4 crimini mushrooms,
small dice
2 tsp balsamic vinegar
1 tsp extra virgin olive oil
2 tsp filtered water

2 lb zucchini, thinly sliced
into noodles
Pinch sea salt
1 Tbsp extra virgin olive oil

¼ cup Parsley Basil Pesto
(page 196)
¼ cup Parmesan cheese, for
garnish

1. Add marinara to a saucepan. Heat on low, covered.

2. For the Italian sausage, combine in a mixing bowl the garlic, oregano, Italian herbs, fennel, rosemary, paprika, black pepper, red pepper flakes if using and salt. Rub mixture with your fingers to bruise the spices.

3. Add the ground turkey, mushrooms, and balsamic vinegar. Mix well.

4. Preheat a nonstick skillet to medium-high. Add the olive oil quickly followed by the turkey sausage. Sauté for 6-8 minutes until lightly browned, breaking up any large clumps. Reduce heat to low and add the water. Partially cover for 3 minutes. Uncover and allow to evaporate for 1 minute. Remove from heat.

5. Preheat a large nonstick pan to medium-high. Add the olive oil, zucchini and a pinch of salt. Sauté, stirring often until zucchini noodles are soft and steaming, 8-10 minutes.

6. Remove from heat and stir in the pesto.

7. Pour into a serving bowl and add the Italian sausage.

8. Serve with the marinara sauce and Parmesan cheese on the side.

SERVES 4

Lutein+Zeaxanthin • 5,232mcg
Omega-3 • 502mg
Vitamin B6 • 65%DV

Spaghetti Squash & Grass-Fed Beef Ragu

1 lb ripe Roma tomatoes, quartered
1 cup filtered water

1 Tbsp extra virgin olive oil
1 medium onion, small dice
1 rib celery, small dice
2 carrots, small dice
3 garlic cloves, minced
1 lb grass-fed ground beef
6 oz can tomato paste
⅓ cup red wine or water
⅓ cup milk, optional
⅛ tsp nutmeg
1 Tbsp dried oregano
1 Tbsp dried Italian herbs

1 tsp evaporated cane sugar
½ tsp sea salt
½ tsp black pepper
Pinch red pepper flakes
1 large spaghetti squash, halved and seeded
2 tsp extra virgin olive oil
¼ cup water

½ cup Italian flat leaf parsley
½ cup grated Parmesan cheese

1. For the ragu, place tomatoes in a high speed blender with the water and puree until smooth.

2. Preheat a large Dutch oven to medium high. Add the oil quickly followed by the onions, celery, carrots, garlic and a pinch of salt. Sauté until the onions are translucent.

3. Add the ground beef. Sauté until the meat is no longer pink. Add the tomato paste. Sauté 2-3 minutes, stirring constantly.

4. Add the wine, stirring and scraping the bottom of the pan to release any brown bits and the wine has evaporated.

5. Turn the heat down to medium low. Add the milk and nutmeg. Allow to mostly evaporate, stirring frequently.

6. Add the pureed tomatoes, oregano, Italian herbs, red pepper flakes, sugar, salt and black pepper.

7. Stir and cover. Allow to simmer 45-60 minutes.

8. Preheat oven to 375°F. Roast the spaghetti squash while simmering the ragu. Drizzle each squash half with olive oil. Place cut-side down in an oven safe baking dish. Add water and bake for 45-60 minutes until the squash is easily pierced with a paring knife. Cool 10 minutes. Using a fork, scrape the squash to create noodles.

9. Stir the parsley into the finished ragu. Serve the noodles with a ladle of ragu. Garnish with Parmesan.

SERVES 4

Lycopene • 14,965mcg
Lutein+Zeaxanthin • 691mcg
Omega-3 • 588mg

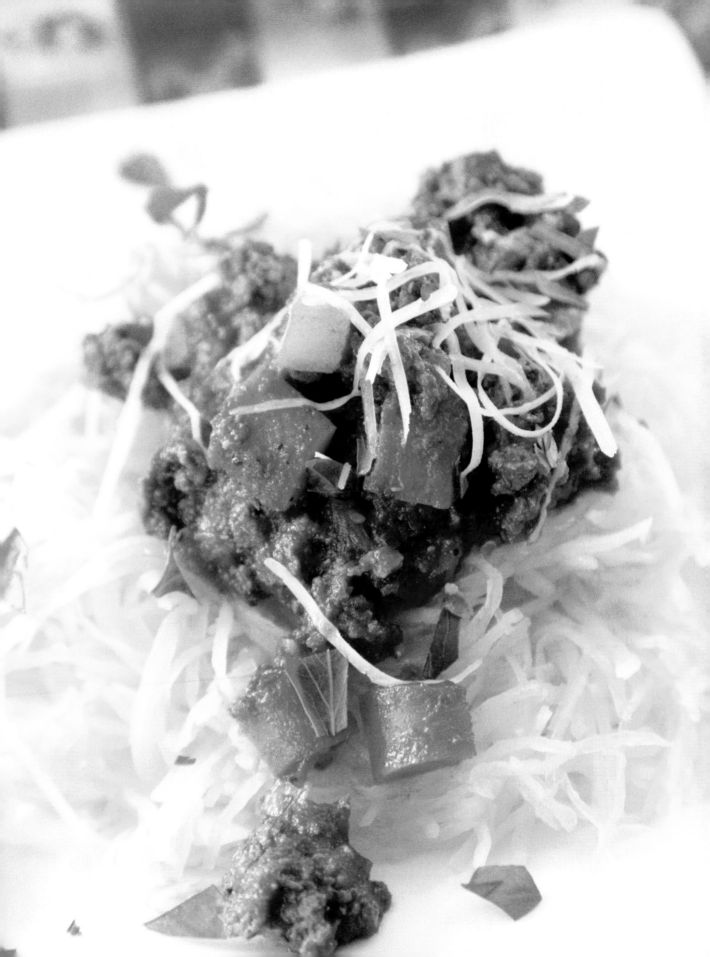

Falafel with Tahini Slaw

15 oz can chickpeas, drained and rinsed

3 Tbsp ground flax seed

⅔ cup fresh Italian flat leaf parsley

¼ cup feta cheese crumbles

1 omega-3 egg

1 tsp lemon zest

1 Tbsp lemon juice

½ tsp sea salt

¼ tsp black pepper

2 Tbsp extra virgin olive oil

12 leaves butter lettuce

1 recipe Rainbow Coleslaw (page 84)

½ recipe Tahini Dip (page 193)

1. To the bowl of a food processor, add chickpeas, flax, parsley, feta, egg, lemon zest and juice, salt and pepper. Process until smooth.

2. Shape into twelve patties.

3. Preheat a non-stick pan to medium. Add half the oil quickly followed by the falafel. Sauté until golden, 5-6 minutes. Flip over and add the remaining Tbsp of olive oil. Sauté an additional 5-6 minutes, until golden.

4. Place each falafel into a butter lettuce leaf to serve.

5. Serve with Tahini Dip and Rainbow Slaw.

SERVES 6

Lutein+Zeaxanthin • 1,486mcg
Omega-3 • 1,004mg
Zinc • 15%DV

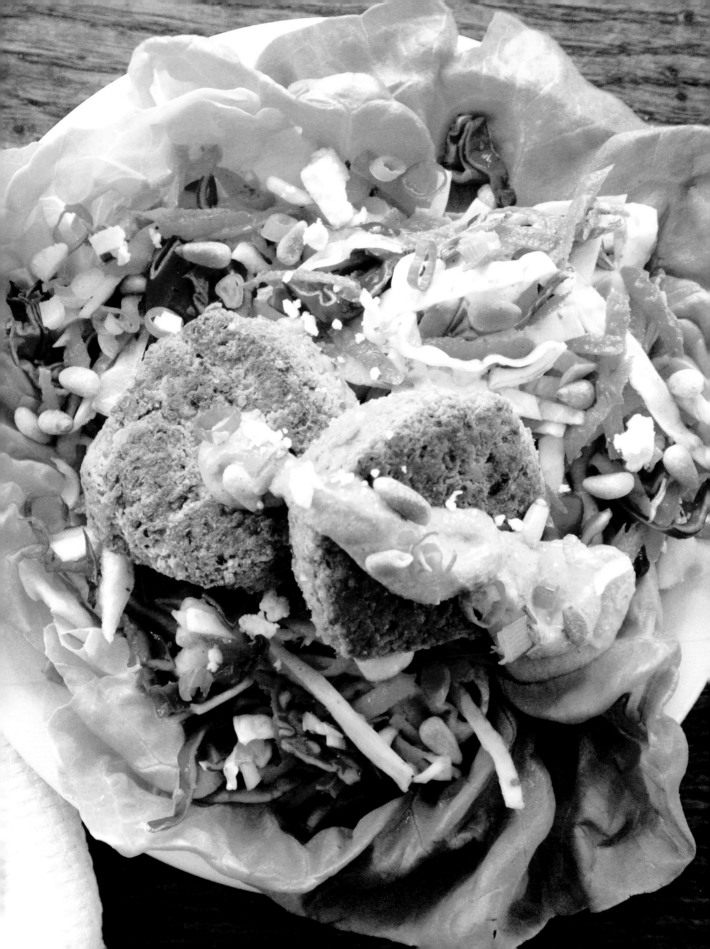

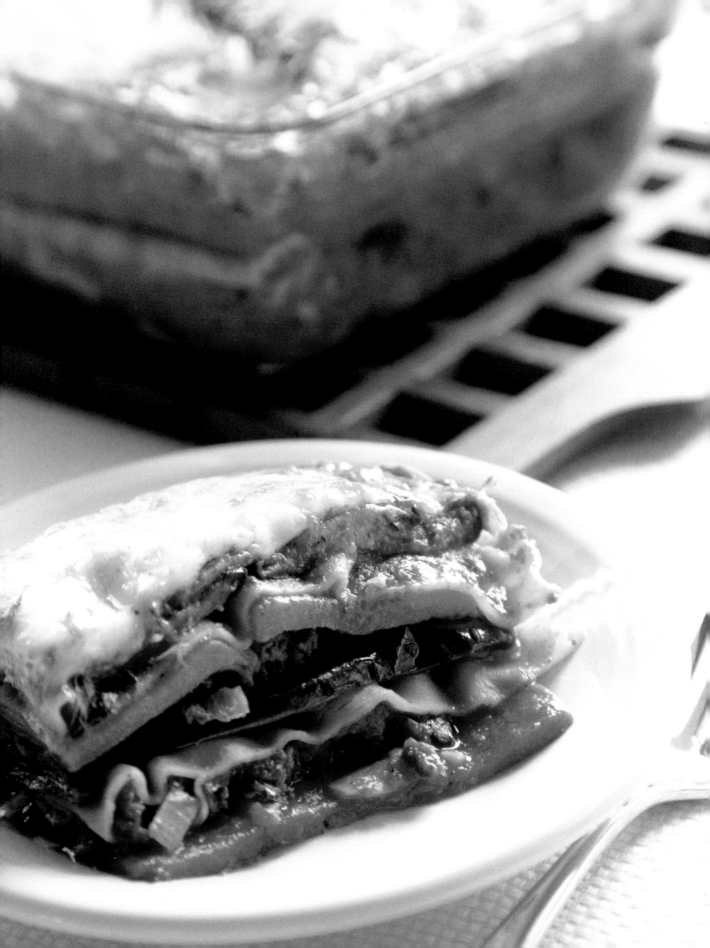

Eggplant Lasagna

2 eggplants, sliced in ⅓"
slices lengthwise
1 Tbsp extra virgin olive oil
Pinch sea salt

1 Tbsp extra virgin olive oil
2 garlic cloves, minced
1 small red onion, diced
¾ lb grass-fed ground beef
or bison
¼ tsp sea salt
¼ tsp black pepper

6 lasagna noodles,
no-boil style

3 bell peppers, roasted,
halved, stems and seeds
removed (page 179)

1 recipe Fresh Marinara
(page 195)
1 cup mozzarella cheese,
grated

1. To roast the eggplant, preheat oven to 375°F. Rub 1 Tbsp olive oil evenly over a baking sheet. Place sliced eggplant on the baking sheet. Flip eggplant over so that a little olive oil is on both sides. Sprinkle with a pinch of salt. Bake for 20-25 minutes until golden brown.

2. For the beef, preheat a sauté pan to medium-high. Add the oil and garlic sautéing briefly followed by the onions, ground beef, salt and pepper.

3. To assemble, lightly grease a 9"×7"×2.5" glass baking dish. Layer in the following order: 1 cup marinara, 2 lasagna noodles, layer of red bell pepper, ½ ground beef, 1 cup marinara, 2 lasagna noodles, layer of eggplant, ½ ground beef, 1 cup marinara, 2 lasagna noodles, layer of orange bell pepper, 1 cup marinara, mozzarella cheese.

4. Preheat oven to 350°F. Bake for 30 minutes covered with aluminum foil. Uncover and finish baking for 20 minutes until cheese is golden and bubbly.

SERVES 8

Peppers may be store-bought or homemade (page 179).

Lycopene • 7,016mcg
Lutein+Zeaxanthin • 354mcg
Zinc • 32%DV

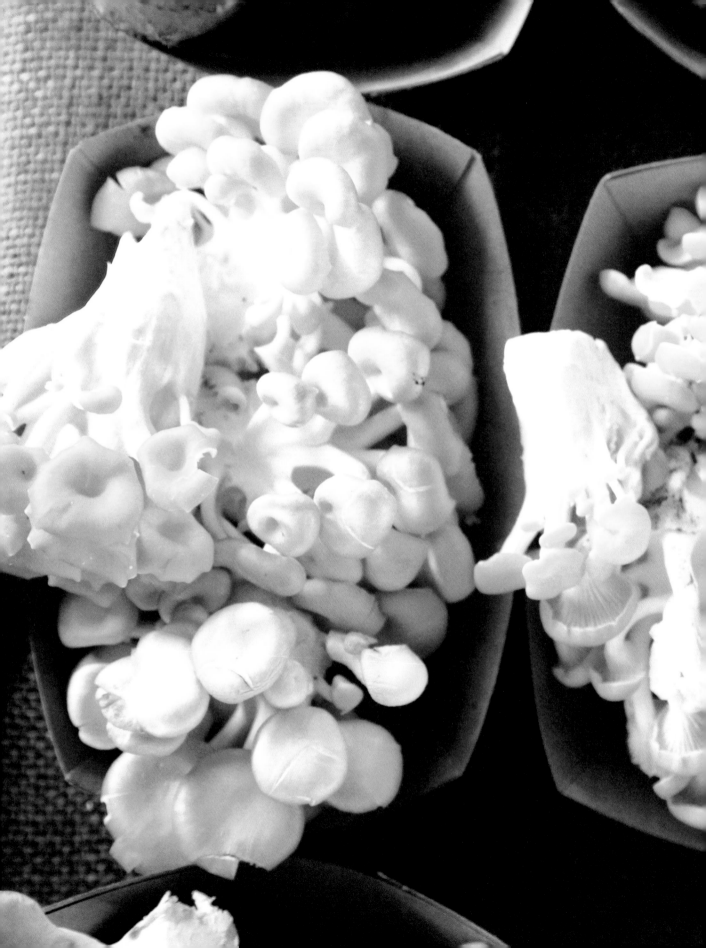

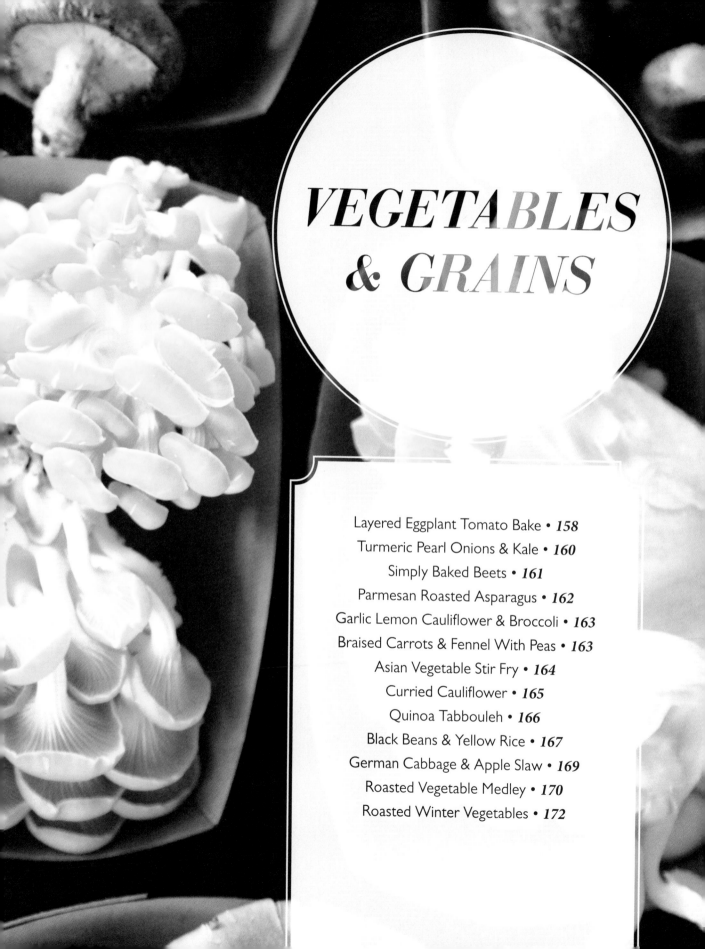

VEGETABLES & GRAINS

Layered Eggplant Tomato Bake

4 tsp extra virgin olive oil
4 ¼" slices red onion, about
   4" diameter
¼ tsp sea salt
¼ tsp black pepper
8 ¼" slices eggplant, about
   4" diameter,
   peeled or unpeeled
2 tsp balsamic vinegar
8 ¼" slices beefsteak
   tomatoes,
   about 4" diameter
1 garlic clove, minced
4 basil leaves, torn or sliced,
   plus more for garnish
¼ cup Parmesan
   or Romano cheese,
   grated

1. Preheat oven to 375°F. Lightly oil an 8"×8" glass baking dish with 1 tsp olive oil.

2. Base layer: 4 onion slices each drizzled with ¼ tsp olive oil

3. Second layer: 4 eggplant slices each drizzled with ¼ tsp balsamic vinegar and a pinch of salt and pepper.

4. Third layer: 4 tomato slices, each drizzled with ¼ tsp olive oil, ¼ clove garlic and torn basil.

5. Fourth layer: 4 eggplant slices, each drizzled with ¼ tsp balsamic vinegar and a pinch of salt and pepper.

6. Top layer: 4 tomato slices, each drizzled with ¼ tsp olive oil and 1 Tbsp cheese.

7. Bake uncovered for 50-60 minutes.

8. Garnish with fresh basil.

SERVES 4

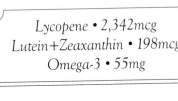

Lycopene • 2,342mcg
Lutein+Zeaxanthin • 198mcg
Omega-3 • 55mg

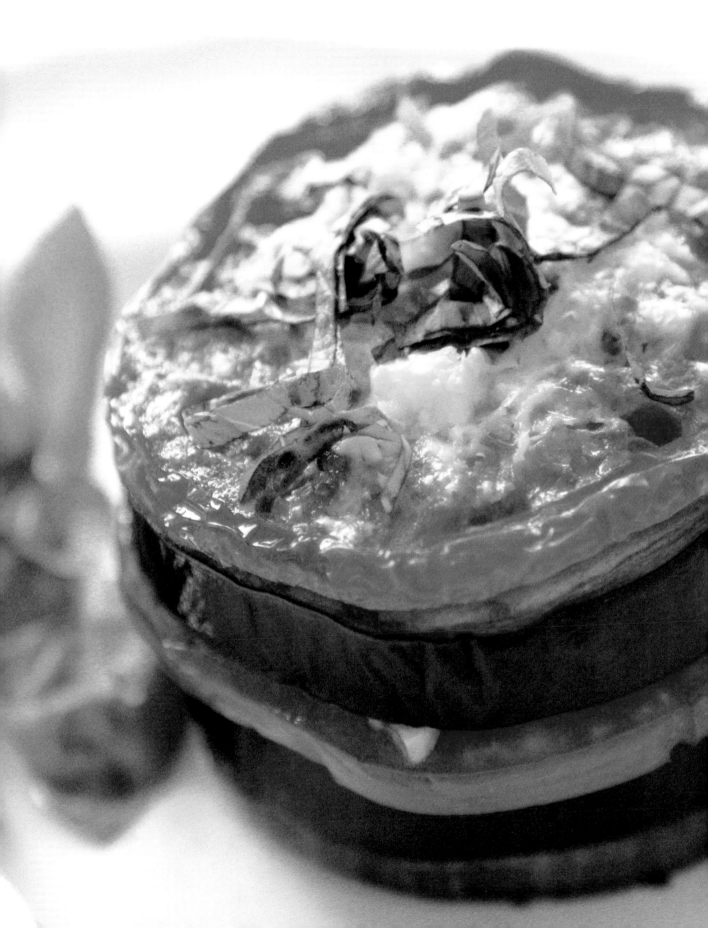

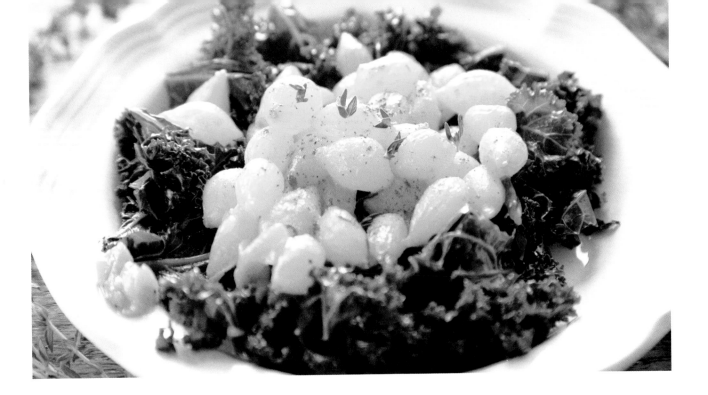

Turmeric Pearl Onions & Kale

16 oz frozen pearl onions, thawed
⅓ cup filtered water
½ cup light coconut milk
¼ tsp sea salt
¼ tsp black pepper

1 tsp fresh thyme
¼ tsp turmeric

1 Tbsp extra virgin olive oil
1 garlic clove, minced
1 bunch kale, ribs removed, diced

2 Tbsp filtered water
¼ tsp sea salt
¼ tsp black pepper

1. For the pearl onions, preheat a skillet to medium. Add the onions and water. Sauté 2-3 minutes.

2. Add the coconut milk, salt, pepper, thyme and turmeric. Reduce the heat and cover. Gently simmer for 15-20 minutes, until creamy.

3. For the kale, preheat a sauté pan to medium. Add the olive oil quickly followed by the garlic, stirring briefly before adding the kale and water. Stir constantly for 2-3 minutes.

4. Turn the heat to medium-low and cover. Stir, as needed, for 5-6 minutes. Lightly season with salt and pepper.

5. To serve, place kale on warmed platter and top with onions.

MAKES 5 CUPS • SERVES 4

Lutein+Zeaxanthin • 26,503mcg
Omega-3 • 149mg
Vitamin C • 144%DV

Simply Baked Beets

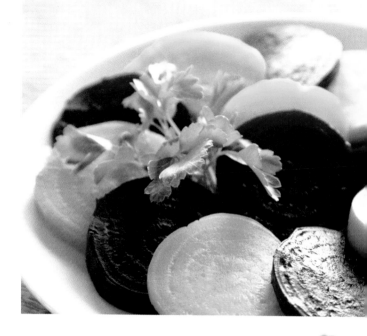

6 beets (golden, red or striped;
    all approximately the same size)

1. Preheat oven to 350°F. Remove greens from beets, if present. Scrub with a vegetable brush under running water to remove any dirt or debris.

2. Wrap each beet in foil and place in a baking dish.

3. Bake for 45 minutes or until tender when pierced with a fork. Remove from oven and allow to cool while still wrapped.

4. Peel the beets under running water by pressing your thumb into the beet, tearing the skin. Allow the water to gently assist. Slice and serve.

SERVES 6

The baking time is dependent on the size of the beet. They are great chilled the next day. Enjoy lightly dressed with the Walnut Oil Vinaigrette (page 176).

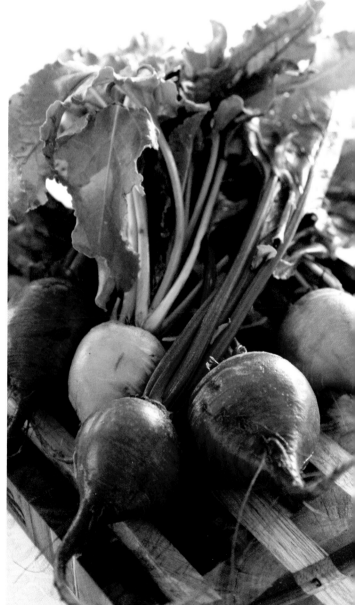

Beta-Carotene • 16mcg
Folate • 22%DV
Zinc • 2%DV

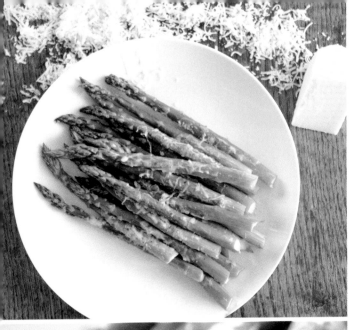

Parmesan Roasted Asparagus

1 lb asparagus
2 Tbsp Avocado Goat
  Cheese Dressing
  (page 177)
1 Tbsp Parmesan cheese,
  grated
⅛ tsp black pepper

1. Preheat oven to 400°F. Snap the woody bottom off of each asparagus stalk.

2. Place on a baking sheet. Brush asparagus stalks with the dressing and sprinkle with cheese. Season with pepper, to taste.

3. Roast in oven for 8-10 minutes, until crisp tender.

SERVES 4

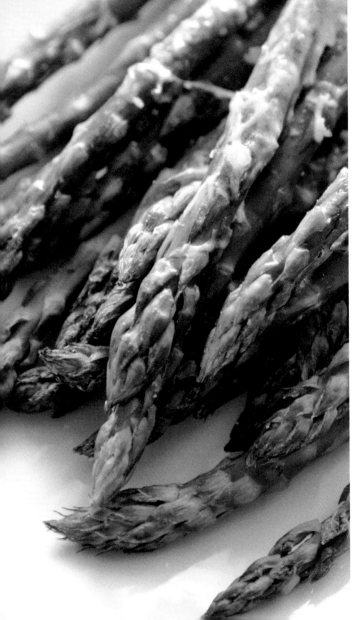

Lutein+Zeaxanthin • 845mcg
Folate • 15%DV
Zinc • 5%DV

Garlic Lemon Cauliflower & Broccoli

1 Tbsp extra virgin olive oil
1 garlic clove, minced
2 cups cauliflower,
   cut into bite-sized florets
2 cups broccoli,
   cut into bite-sized florets
¼ cup water or stock of
   choice

1 Tbsp lemon juice
⅛ tsp lemon zest
 Pinch sea salt
⅛ tsp black pepper

1. Preheat a heavy lidded skillet to medium. Add the olive oil and garlic quickly followed by the cauliflower and broccoli. Sauté for 3 minutes, stirring constantly.

2. Reduce the heat to medium-low. Add the stock and cover. Steam for 6-8 minutes until the broccoli and cauliflower are crisp tender.

3. Remove from the heat and stir in the lemon juice and zest. Season with a pinch of salt and pepper.

SERVES 8

Lutein+Zeaxanthin • 656mcg
Folate • 15%DV
Vitamin C • 113%DV

Braised Carrots & Fennel with Peas

1 Tbsp extra virgin olive oil
3 large carrots,
   cut into wedges
1 large fennel bulb,
   cored and sliced
1 tsp fresh ginger, grated
⅓ cup water or stock of
   choice
1 cup frozen peas
 Pinch sea salt
¼ tsp black pepper

1. Preheat a sauté pan to medium. Add the oil quickly followed by the carrots and fennel. Stir frequently for 2-3 minutes.

2. Add the ginger and water or stock, reduce heat to low and cover. Cook until crisp tender, 7-10 minutes.

3. Remove from the heat and add the frozen peas, salt and pepper. Cover and allow to sit for 5 minutes before serving.

SERVES 4

Substitute the juice of ½ an orange for part of the water or stock, if desired.

Vitamin A • 171%DV
Lutein+Zeaxanthin • 1,077mcg
Vitamin C • 23%DV

Asian Vegetable Stir Fry

3 Tbsp water
3 Tbsp soy sauce or tamari
1 Tbsp arrowroot starch

1 Tbsp extra virgin olive oil
2 garlic cloves, finely minced
2 tsp fresh ginger, grated
1 Thai chili, finely minced, optional
1 small onion, diced
1 orange bell pepper, diced
1 large carrot, sliced
8 shiitake mushrooms, stems removed, sliced
1 cup snow peas
3 cups Napa cabbage, quartered, cored and sliced into ¼" strips

1. In a small bowl, stir together water, soy sauce or tamari and the arrowroot starch. Set aside.

2. Preheat a 12" skillet or wok to medium-high. Add oil quickly followed by the garlic, ginger, Thai chili if using, onion, bell pepper and carrot. Sauté 4-6 minutes, stirring often, until the vegetables begin to soften.

3. Next add the mushrooms, snow peas and Napa cabbage. Sauté and stir until cabbage begins to wilt.

4. Add the soy sauce mixture and cook until thickened. Serve hot.

SERVES 6

Beta-Carotene • 1,515mcg
Vitamin C • 93%DV
Zinc • 4%DV

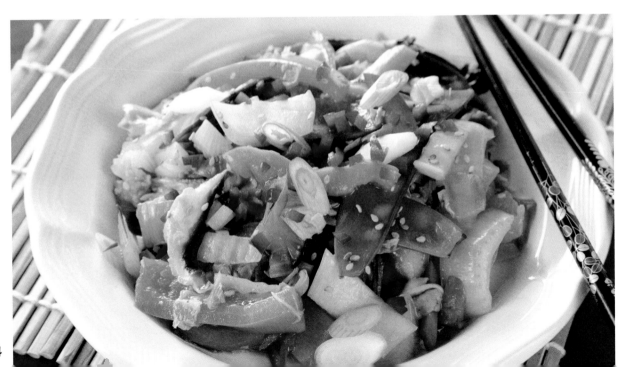

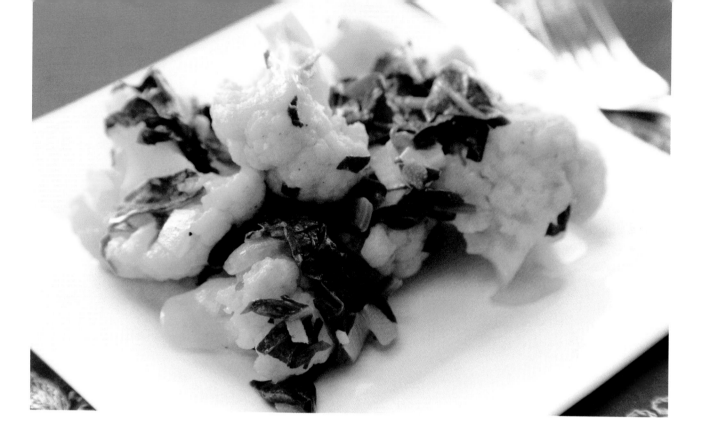

Curried Cauliflower

1 Tbsp extra virgin olive oil
1 sweet onion, small dice
2 garlic cloves, minced
2 tsp fresh ginger, grated
¼ tsp red pepper flakes
¼ tsp black pepper
¼ tsp sea salt
½ tsp ground coriander
½ tsp ground cumin
½ tsp turmeric
¾ cup light coconut milk
1 head cauliflower, cut into bite-sized florets
2 cups fresh spinach, roughly chopped

1. Preheat a large lidded sauce pan to medium. Add oil quickly followed by the onion and a pinch of salt. Sauté for 5-6 minutes until onion is soft and begins to take on color.

2. Add the garlic, ginger, red pepper flakes, black pepper, salt, coriander, cumin and turmeric.

3. Stir in the coconut milk and cauliflower. Reduce heat to medium-low. Cover and simmer for 15-20 minutes until the cauliflower is tender.

4. Stir in spinach until just wilted. Serve hot.

MAKES 6 CUPS • SERVES 4

Lutein+Zeaxanthin • 2,355mcg
Omega-3 • 108mg
Vitamin C • 127%DV

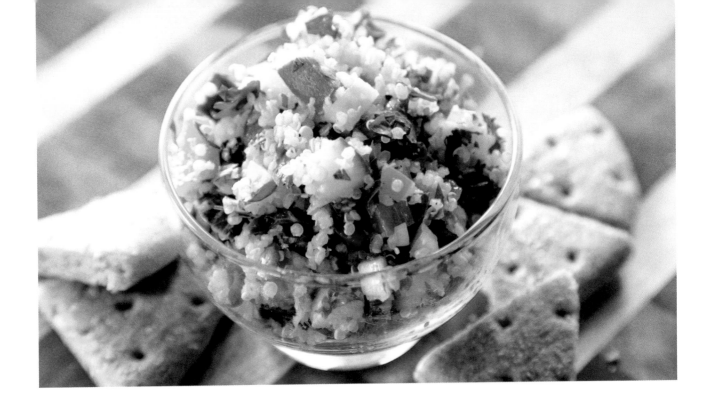

Quinoa Tabbouleh

½ medium red onion, small dice

½ orange bell pepper, small dice

1 cup Persian cucumbers, small dice

1 jalapeño, seeded and ribs removed, finely diced

1 ½ cup Italian flat leaf parsley, chopped

⅓ cup tomato, small dice

2 garlic cloves, minced

¼ cup extra virgin olive oil

2 Tbsp lemon juice

¼ tsp sea salt

¼ tsp black pepper

2 cups cooked quinoa (see directions to right)

1. Place all ingredients in a mixing bowl and stir to combine.

2. Serve or store refrigerated up to 3 days.

SERVES 4

The ancient grain quinoa is a source of complete protein.

Lutein+Zeaxanthin • 1,308mcg
Vitamin C • 109%DV
Zinc • 10%DV

How to Cook Quinoa

1 cup quinoa, rinsed and drained   1 ¼ cups water   ½ tsp sea salt

1. Add quinoa, water and salt to a medium sauce pan, bring to a simmer over medium-high heat.

2. Reduce heat to low. Stir and cover. Cook 12-15 minutes.

3. Remove from the heat. Cool covered 10-15 minutes.

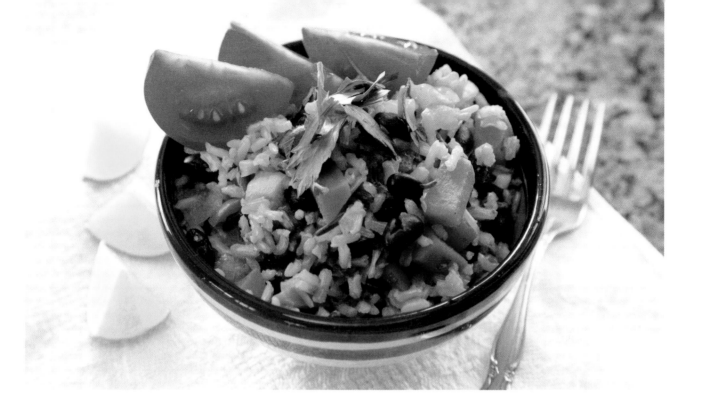

Black Beans & Yellow Rice

1 Tbsp extra virgin olive oil
1 garlic clove, minced
½ cup onion, finely diced
½ cup orange bell pepper, small dice
1 cup sweet potato, small dice
1 can black beans, drained and rinsed

½ tsp sea salt
½ tsp turmeric
2¼ cups water or stock of choice
1 cup wild rice medley (can be substituted with brown or red rice)

½ cup scallions, sliced

1. Preheat a 4½ quart covered sauce pan to medium-high. Add oil quickly followed by the garlic, onions, bell pepper, sweet potato and black beans. Sauté for 2-3 minutes.

2. Add salt, turmeric, water or stock and rice. Stir and bring to a boil.

3. Reduce the heat to low and cover. Simmer 40-50 minutes.

4. Remove from heat. Allow the rice to rest 10 minutes, covered.

5. Stir in the scallions and serve.

SERVES 6

For a little heat, consider serving with roasted chili peppers.

Beta-Carotene • 2,339mcg
Vitamin C • 57%DV
Vitamin E • 6%DV

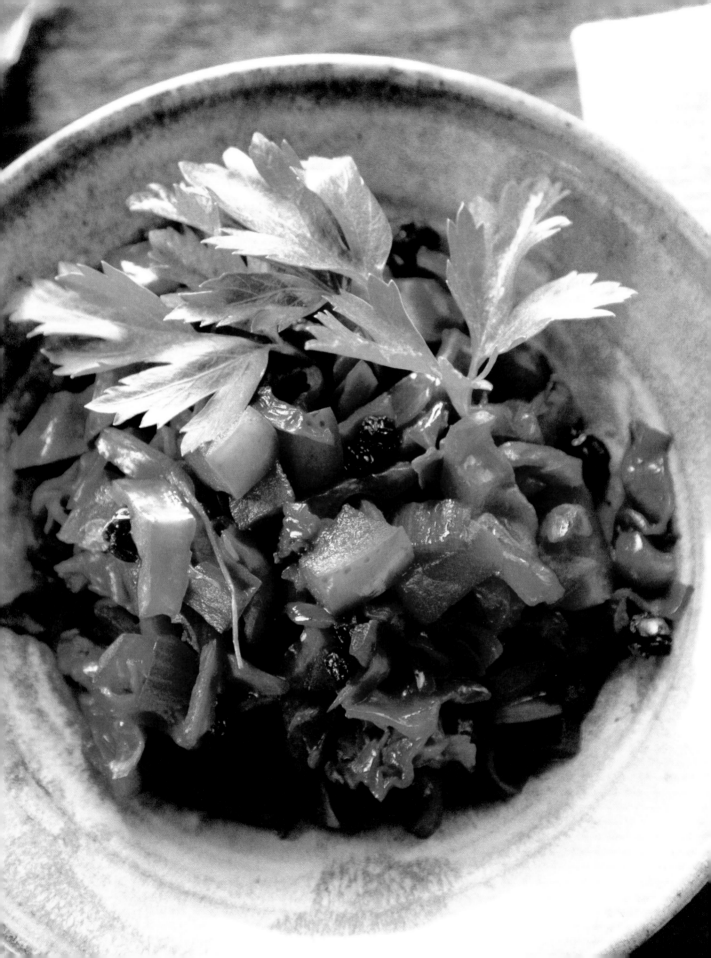

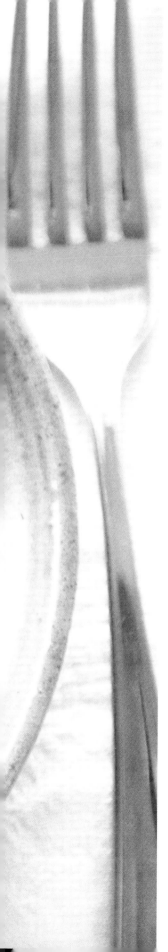

German Cabbage & Apple Slaw

1 small red cabbage
⅓ cup malt vinegar
1 Tbsp evaporated cane sugar
½ tsp sea salt

1 Tbsp extra virgin olive oil
1 organic apple (e.g., Fuji or Macintosh), ½" dice
1 cup sweet onion, diced
2 Tbsp organic raisins or currants
3 whole cloves pierced into 1" chunk of carrot
1 bay leaf
2¼ cups boiling water
¼ cup red wine or water

1. Remove any tough outer leaves of the cabbage and cut into quarters. Remove the core. Shred the cabbage, slicing the quarters crosswise into ¼" strips.

2. Place the shredded cabbage in a large mixing bowl. Add vinegar, sugar, and salt. Stir well to evenly coat the cabbage. Allow cabbage to sit while preparing the apples and onions.

3. Preheat a nonreactive large Dutch oven to medium. Add the oil quickly followed by the apple and onion, stirring frequently for 5 minutes.

4. Add the cabbage, currants, clove-studded carrot and bay leaf. Pour the boiling water over the cabbage along with the wine; stir.

5. Reduce the heat to low. Cover and simmer for 1 hour, stirring occasionally.

6. Remove the carrot. Serve hot or at room temperature.

SERVES 4

Lutein+Zeaxanthin • 492mcg
Omega-3 • 111mg
Vitamin C • 143%DV

Roasted Vegetable Medley

1 medium red onion,
  ¾" wedges
1 large beet, ¾" wedges
3 medium carrots,
  ½" wedges
½ lb Brussels sprouts, halved
2 cups sweet potato,
  ¾" dice
1½ Tbsp extra virgin olive oil
¼ tsp sea salt

1 garlic clove, finely minced
¼ cup Parmesan
  or Romano cheese
¼ tsp black pepper
¼ tsp sea salt
2 tsp fresh rosemary
1 Tbsp fresh oregano
1 Tbsp Italian
  flat leaf parsley

*In a pinch, you can use dried
herbs to replace fresh.*

1. For the roasted vegetables, preheat oven to 400°F. Add onion, beets, carrots, Brussels sprouts and sweet potato to a mixing bowl.

2. Drizzle with olive oil and ¼ tsp salt. Stir to ensure an even coating of oil. Place vegetables in a 10"×15" glass baking dish.

3. Roast for 40-50 minutes, stirring 1-2 times for even browning. Remove vegetables from the oven when tender.

4. Combine garlic, cheese, pepper, salt, rosemary, oregano and parsley. Rub the mixture between your fingers to bring out the flavors of the herbs.

5. Sprinkle vegetables with herb and cheese mixture. Return to the oven for 5 minutes.

SERVES 6

Vitamin A • 235%DV
Lutein+Zeaxanthin • 26,502mcg
Vitamin C • 63%DV

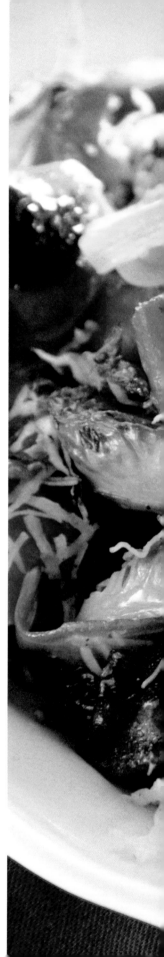

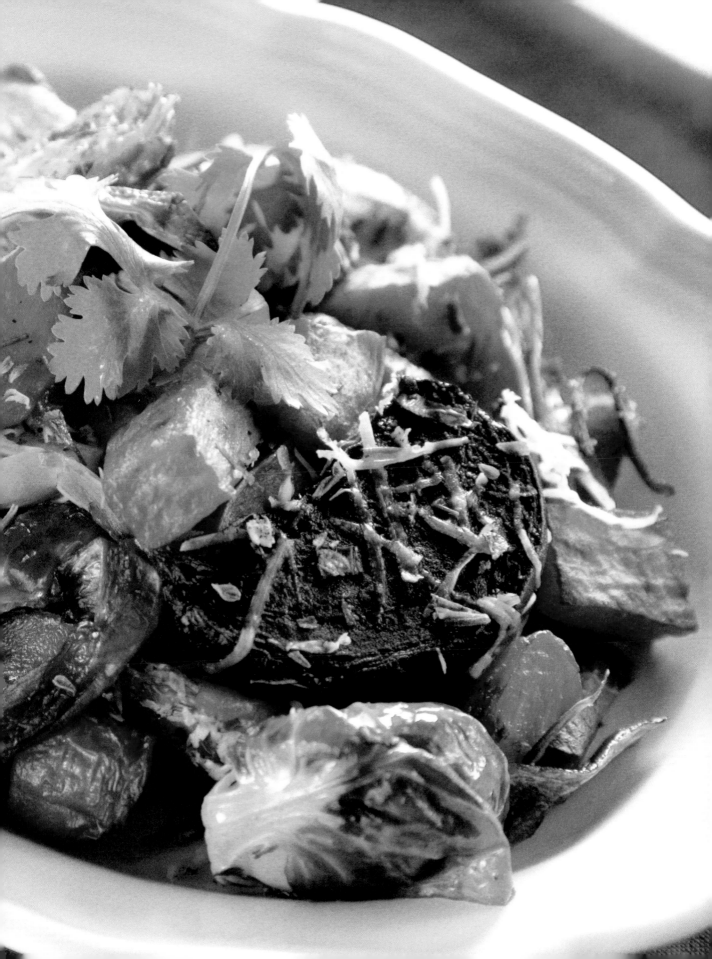

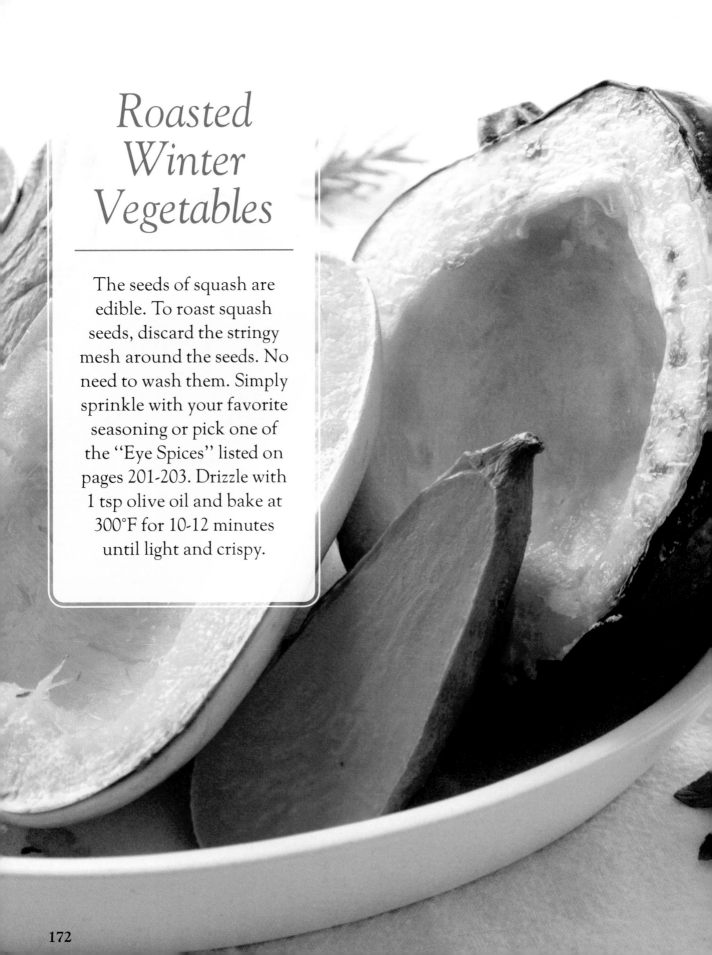

Roasted Winter Vegetables

The seeds of squash are edible. To roast squash seeds, discard the stringy mesh around the seeds. No need to wash them. Simply sprinkle with your favorite seasoning or pick one of the "Eye Spices" listed on pages 201-203. Drizzle with 1 tsp olive oil and bake at 300°F for 10-12 minutes until light and crispy.

Butternut Squash, 2½ lb

1. Halve lengthwise.

2. Scrape out the seeds and strings using a spoon.

3. Rub the cut sides with 1 tsp olive oil. Place cut side down in a glass baking dish.

4. Bake for at 350°F for 45-55 minutes, until tender and easily pierced with a paring knife.

SERVES 4

Beta-Carotene • 11,832mcg

Acorn or Kobacha Squash, 1 lb

1. Halve lengthwise.

2. Scrape out the seeds and strings using a spoon.

3. Rub cut sides with 1 tsp olive oil. Place cut side down in a glass baking dish.

4. Bake at 350°F for 40-60 minutes until tender and easily pierced with a paring knife.

SERVES 4

Lutein+Zeaxanthin • 41mcg

Spaghetti Squash, 2½ lb

1. Cut in half lengthwise.

2. Scrape out the seeds and strings using a spoon.

3. Rub the cut sides with 1 tsp olive oil.

4. Add ¼ cup water to a glass baking dish. Place the squash cut side down, roast at 375°F for 45-60 minutes until tender and easily pierced with a paring knife.

5. Allow to cool 10 minutes in the baking dish. Using a fork, scrape the inside to create the spaghetti noodles.

SERVES 4

Omega-3 • 426mg

Sweet Potato, 4 Potatoes

1. Scrub the potatoes clean.

2. On a baking sheet, poke 2-3 holes with a knife or cut a small slice from one end to allow steam to escape.

3. Bake at 375°F for 40-60 minutes depending on size. The sweet potato will be soft when pierced.

SERVES 4

Beta-Carotene • 15,883mcg

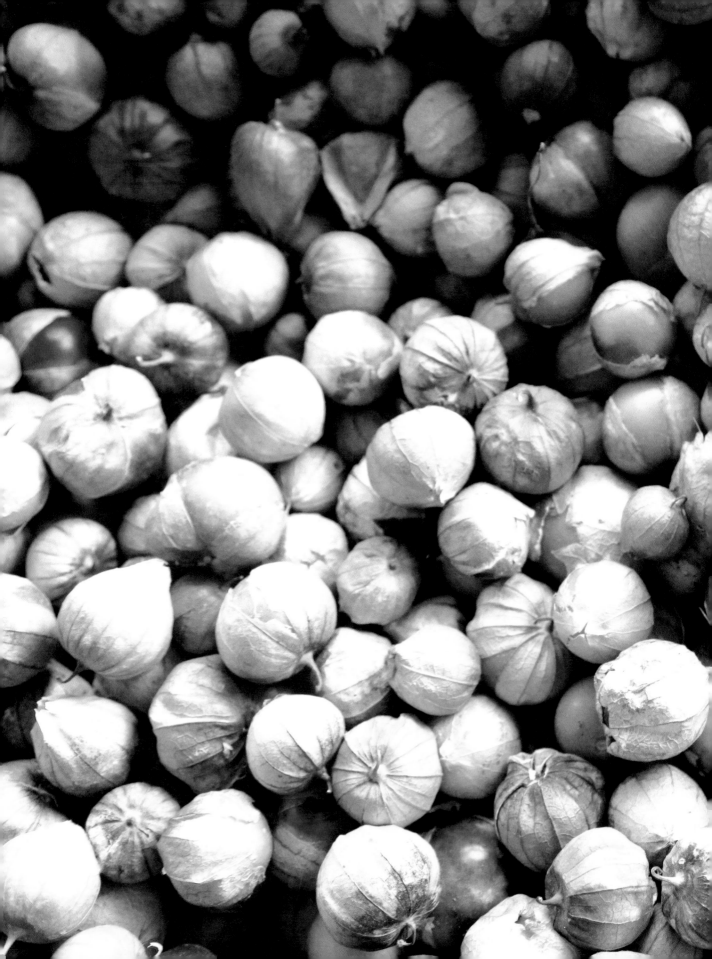

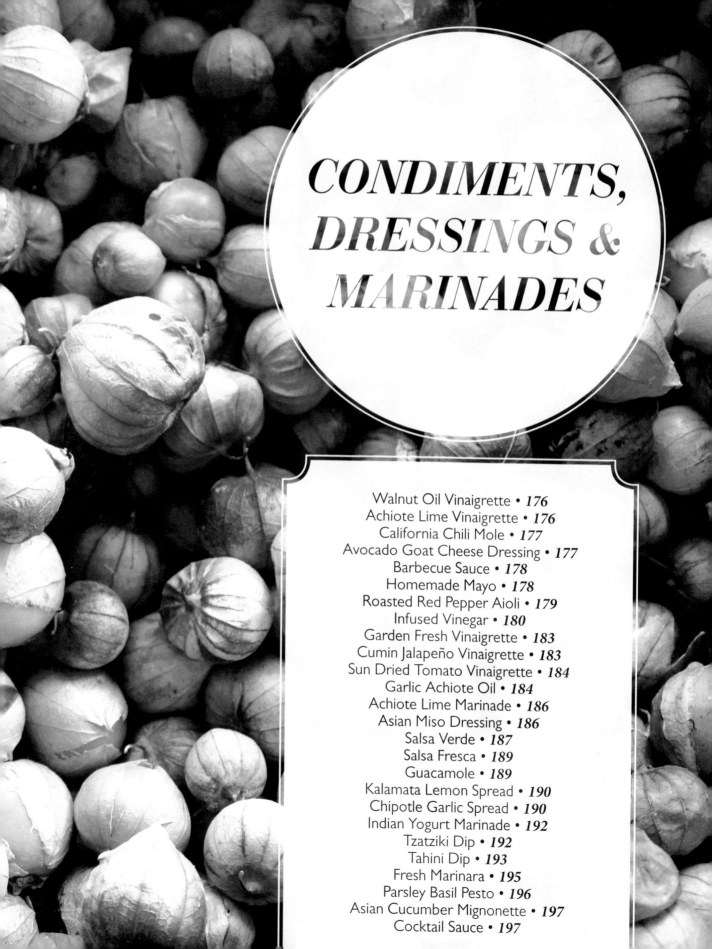

CONDIMENTS, DRESSINGS & MARINADES

Walnut Oil Vinaigrette

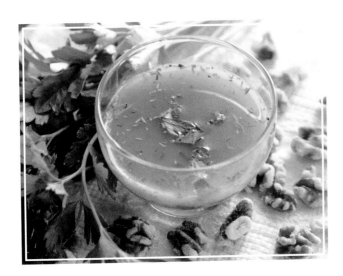

3 large anchovy fillets, mashed
1 garlic clove, minced with a garlic press
2 tsp whole grain mustard
1 tsp dried bouquet garni
¼ tsp black pepper
3 Tbsp apple cider vinegar
2 Tbsp walnut oil
3 Tbsp extra virgin olive oil

1. Combine anchovies, garlic, mustard, bouquet garni and black pepper with the vinegar.

2. Whisk in the walnut and olive oils.

3. Keep stored in a sealed container in the refrigerator for up to 3 days.

MAKES ⅔ CUP • SERVES 7

Beta-Carotene • 5mcg
Omega-3 • 363mg
Vitamin E • 3%DV

Achiote Lime Vinaigrette

3 Tbsp lime juice
3 Tbsp Garlic Achiote Oil (page 184)
1 Tbsp garlic, minced
¼ tsp sea salt
¼ tsp black pepper
1 tsp Mexican oregano
¼ tsp ground cumin

1. Whisk to combine all ingredients.

2. Keep refrigerated for up to 7 days.

Lutein+Zeaxanthin • 2mcg
Omega-3 • 44mg
Vitamin E • 4%DV

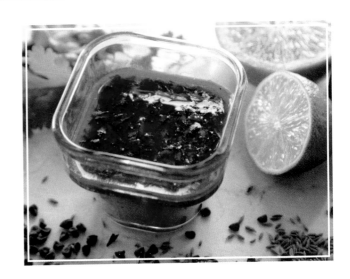

MAKES ½ CUP • SERVES 8

California Chili Mole

1 cup boiling water
1 oz dried California mild chilies; ribs and seeds removed, broken into pieces
1 tsp achiote seeds
2 tsp cacao nibs
2 garlic cloves, coarsely chopped
1 Tbsp maple syrup or raw honey
1 Tbsp apple cider vinegar or lime juice
1 Tbsp extra virgin olive oil
2 Tbsp pepita seeds
½ tsp sea salt
¼ tsp black pepper

1. Place all ingredients into a high-speed blender. Puree until smooth.

2. Keep refrigerated in an airtight container for up to 1 week.

MAKES 1½ CUPS • SERVES 10

Marinate fish or chicken and grill. Use as condiment for brown rice, pasta or tofu. Freeze extra as ice cubes.

Beta-Carotene • 52mcg
Vitamin B6 • 12%DV
Zinc • 4%DV

Avocado Goat Cheese Dressing

6 oz goat cheese
1 garlic clove, minced
3 scallions, sliced
1 ripe avocado
¼ tsp black pepper
¼ tsp sea salt
1 Tbsp lemon juice
2 Tbsp tarragon vinegar
1 shallot, minced, about ¼ cup
½ cup baby spinach, lightly packed*
⅓ cup filtered water, divided
3 Tbsp fresh parsley, chopped

1. Place all ingredients except 2 Tbsp water and parsley into a food processor.

2. Blend until smooth. Add water 1 Tbsp at a time until desired consistency is reached.

3. Add parsley and pulse 2-3 times until combined.

4. Store refrigerated in an airtight container for up to 5 days.

*or romaine, Swiss chard, red leaf, mustard greens

MAKES 2 CUPS • SERVES 12

Beta-Carotene • 146mcg
Lutein+Zeaxanthin • 264mcg
Omega-3 • 15mg

Barbecue Sauce

2 Tbsp extra virgin olive oil, divided

½ large onion, ½" dice

2 garlic cloves, crushed

6 oz can tomato paste

1 large roasted bell pepper (page 179)

2 Tbsp cacao nibs soaked in ¼ cup hot filtered water for 10-15 minutes

⅓ cup red wine vinegar

2 tsp Worcestershire sauce

2 tsp smoked paprika

1 Tbsp dried oregano

2 tsp dried rosemary

¼ tsp cayenne pepper, to taste

1 Tbsp molasses

¼ tsp sea salt

¼ tsp black pepper

2 Tbsp red wine or water, to adjust consistency

Lycopene • 4,027mcg
Lutein+Zeaxanthin • 59mcg
Vitamin C • 36%DV

1. In a skillet preheated to medium. Add 1 Tbsp olive oil quickly followed by the onions and garlic. Sauté for 1-2 minutes.

2. Add the tomato paste. Sauté 2-3 minutes, stirring frequently. Remove from the heat.

3. Place into a high-speed blender with all remaining ingredients. Puree until smooth.

4. If the sauce is too thick, add water or red wine 1 Tbsp at a time to achieve desired consistency.

MAKES 3 CUPS • SERVES 12

Homemade Mayo

1 omega-3 egg, hard boiled, yolk only

1 whole omega-3 egg, hard boiled

1 tsp mustard, Dijon-style

⅛ tsp cayenne pepper

½ tsp evaporated cane sugar

½ tsp sea salt

½ cup extra virgin olive oil or canola oil, divided

¼ cup plain Greek yogurt, non- or low-fat

1 Tbsp lemon juice

Certain brands of Greek yogurt contain higher amounts of protein than others. Aim for the highest protein to sugar ratio available.

Lutein+Zeaxanthin • 19mcg
Omega-3 • 66mg
Vitamin E • 4%DV

A high speed blender is required for this recipe to emulsify to a spreadable consistency.

1. Place egg, egg yolk, mustard, cayenne pepper, sugar, salt and ¼ cup of oil into a high speed blender. Puree until well blended.

2. Add the yogurt and lemon juice. Puree until smooth.

3. With the blender running, drizzle in the final ¼ cup oil and puree until thickened.

MAKES 1¼ CUPS • 20 SERVINGS

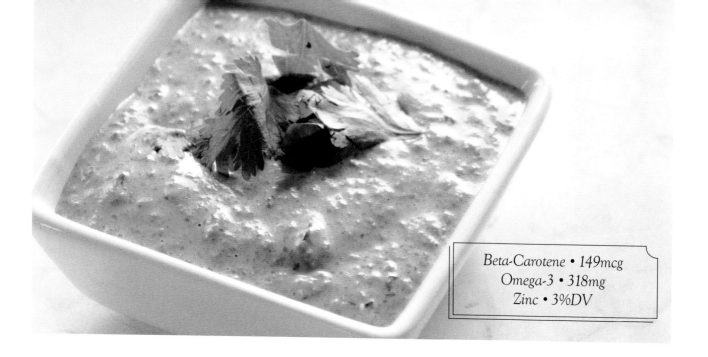

Beta-Carotene • 149mcg
Omega-3 • 318mg
Zinc • 3%DV

Roasted Red Pepper Aioli

Homemade Roasted Bell Peppers

For an electric broiler, preheat to highest setting. Place bell peppers on a baking sheet. Roast under the broiler so that peppers are approximately 3" from the heat source. Char the skins on all sides. Remove from oven. *For a gas stove top*, turn burner to high. Place bell pepper on top of the grate, turning as needed to char the skin on all sides.

Place in a glass bowl. Cover the bowl with plastic wrap. Cover with a towel to retain heat. Allow to sit 15-30 minutes. Peel the charred skin away, rinsing under running water as needed. Remove ribs and seeds.

½ cup roasted bell pepper, roughly chopped
⅓ cup Homemade Mayo (page 178) or organic store-bought mayonnaise
1 garlic clove, finely minced
2 tsp lemon juice
2 tsp ground flax seed
3 Tbsp parsley or cilantro, minced
¼ tsp sea salt
¼ tsp black pepper

1. Combine all ingredients in a blender or mini food chopper. Puree until smooth.

2. Store in the refrigerator sealed for up to 3 days.

MAKES 1½ CUPS • SERVES 16

Infused Vinegar

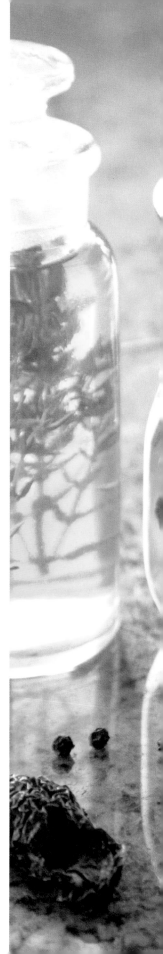

4 cups vinegar (such as rice, apple cider, red wine, champagne)

fresh herbs
⅔ cup basil
3-4 sprigs rosemary
2-3 sprigs oregano
2-3 sprigs tarragon

spices & flavors
5-10 whole black peppercorns
1-2 Thai chilies
2-3 garlic cloves
4-6 sun dried tomatoes
2-3 dried Ancho chilies
10 goji berries

Sterilized jars with non-metallic lids

1. To sterilize jars, completely submerge jars and lids in a pot of water. Over medium heat, bring water to a gentle boil. Boil for 10 minutes.

2. Choose your favorite vinegar.

3. Choose your favorite herbs, one or more. Clean and pat herbs dry. Rub or twist the herbs to release their essential oil. Place clean herbs into a sterilized jar.

4. Choose your spices and flavors and add to a jar.

5. Heat the vinegar of your choice to a simmer, at least 190°F. Carefully pour the vinegar over the herbs and spices to completely submerge. Tightly cover the jar with a non-metallic lid to seal (e.g., wine bottle with a cork) Allow to steep at room temperature for 7-10 days.

6. Strain the vinegar through a fine mesh into sterilized bottles that seal. Refrigerate up to 1 month.

MAKES 1 QUART

Makes a great gift!

Nutrient content will vary with herbs and spices used. See pages 224-225 for more information.

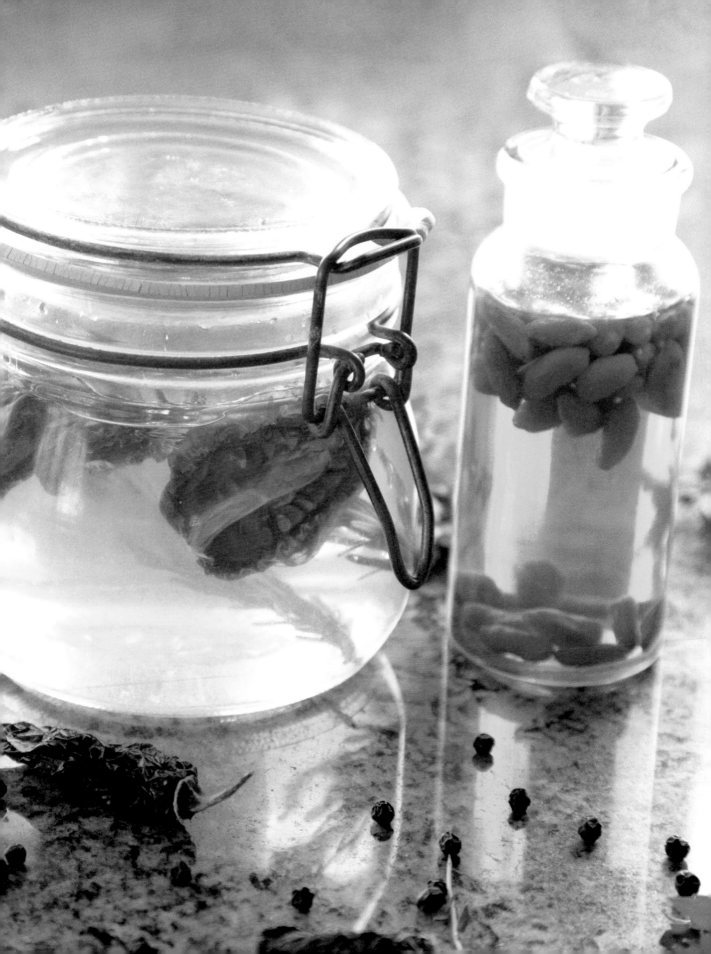

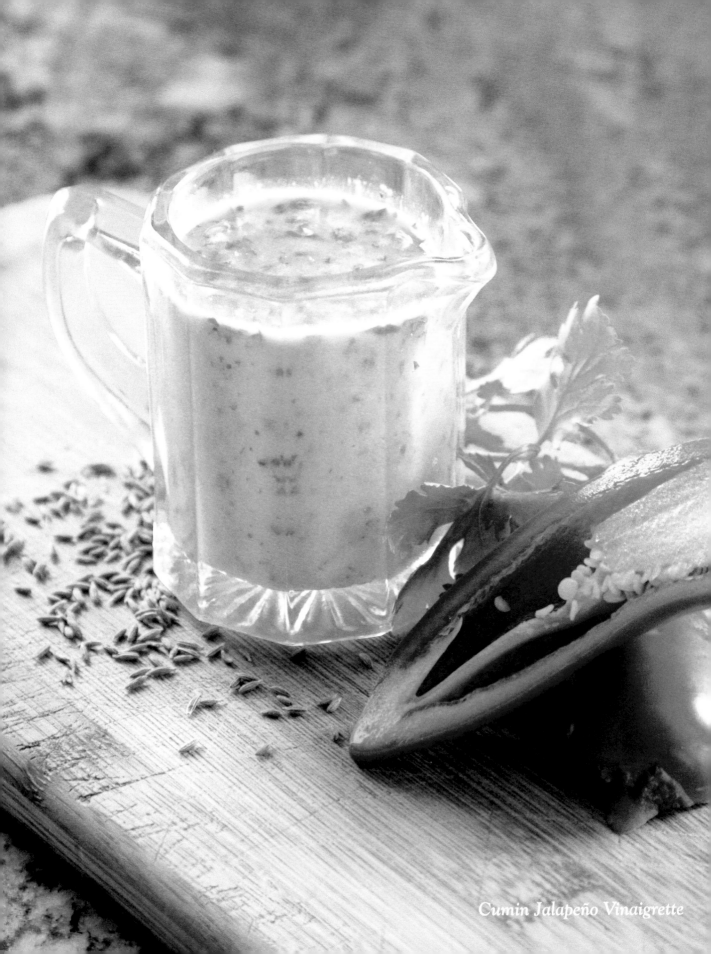

Cumin Jalapeño Vinaigrette

Garden Fresh Vinaigrette

1 orange bell pepper,
  roughly chopped
1 garlic clove, minced
½ cup shallot,
  roughly chopped
1 Tbsp Dijon style mustard
3 Tbsp tarragon vinegar
¼ tsp sea salt
¼ tsp black pepper, to taste
3 radishes, coarsely
  chopped
¼ cup cucumber, diced
¼ cup extra virgin olive oil

1. Place ingredients except olive oil into a blender and puree.

2. Slowly stream in olive oil while blender is running to emulsify.

3. Keep refrigerated for up to 3 days.

MAKES 2 CUPS • SERVES 16

Beta-Carotene • 229mcg
Omega-3 • 140mg
Vitamin C • 31%DV

Cumin Jalapeño Vinaigrette

1 jalapeño, ribs and seeds
  removed, roughly chopped
1 garlic clove, crushed
2 tsp whole grain mustard
2 Tbsp lime juice
2 Tbsp red wine vinegar
1 Tbsp agave nectar
  or raw honey
½ tsp ground cumin
¼ tsp sea salt
¼ tsp black pepper
¼ cup extra virgin olive oil
3 Tbsp cilantro, chopped

1. Place all ingredients except cilantro into a blender and puree. Add cilantro and pulse to incorporate.

2. Keep refrigerated for up to 7 days.

MAKES 1 CUP • SERVES 12

Lutein+Zeaxanthin • 11mcg
Omega-3 • 47mg
Vitamin E • 4%DV

Sun Dried Tomato Vinaigrette

2 Roma tomatoes,
   quartered
2 Tbsp red onion, small dice
1 garlic clove, minced
3 Tbsp tarragon vinegar
2 Tbsp filtered water
¼ cup extra virgin olive oil
¼ tsp sea salt
¼ tsp black pepper
8 kalamata olives,
   pitted and finely minced
2 Tbsp sun dried tomatoes,
   finely minced

1. Place the fresh tomatoes, onions, garlic, vinegar, water, olive oil, salt and pepper into a high-speed blender.

2. Puree until smooth.

3. Transfer the mixture into a serving dish and stir in the finely minced olives and sun dried tomatoes.

4. Keep refrigerated in an airtight container for up to 1 week.

MAKES 1½ CUPS • 12 SERVINGS

Lycopene • 649mcg
Omega-3 • 63mg
Zinc • 10%DV

Garlic Achiote Oil

¾ cup expeller pressed
   canola oil
3 Tbsp achiote seeds
2 garlic cloves,
   lightly crushed

1. Add the oil, achiote seeds and garlic to a sauce pan. Turn the heat to low to very gently heat the oil.

2. Look for little bubbles to form around the garlic. In 10-15 minutes, the oil will turn a deep reddish orange color.

3. Remove from the heat and allow to cool in the sauce pan.

4. Strain and keep refrigerated for up to 2 weeks.

MAKES ¾ CUP

Achiote/Annatto is high in Zeaxanthin and Vitamin E. See page 233 for details.

Omega-3 • 52mg

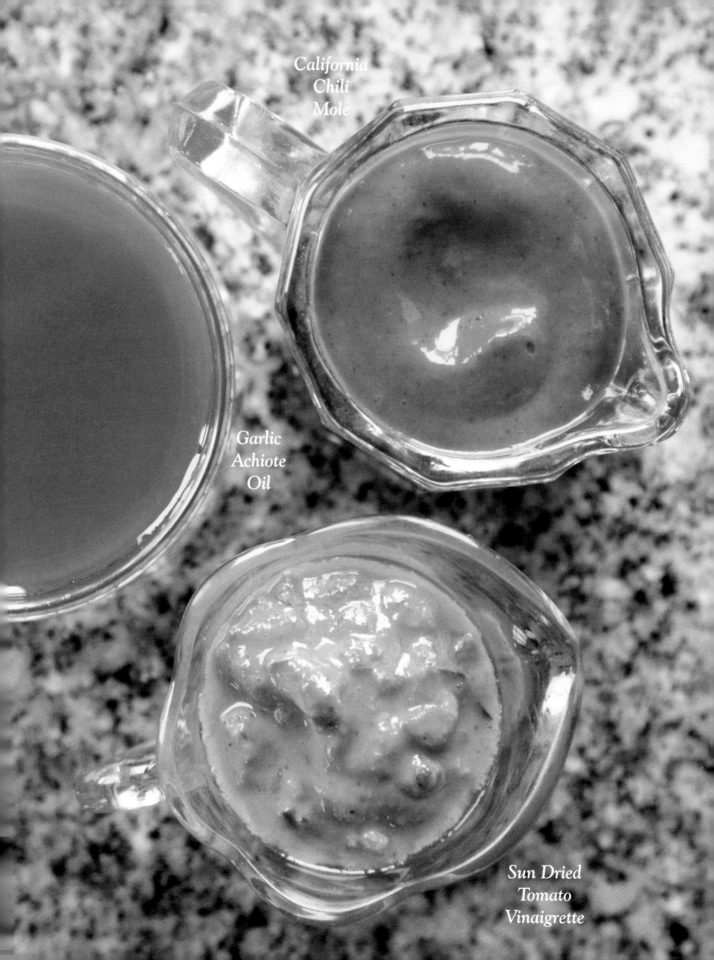

California
Chili
Mole

Garlic
Achiote
Oil

Sun Dried
Tomato
Vinaigrette

Achiote Lime Marinade

1 Tbsp achiote seeds
¼ tsp cumin seeds
2 tsp Mexican oregano
2 garlic cloves, minced
¼ tsp ground allspice
¼ tsp sea salt
¼ tsp black pepper
2 Tbsp bitter orange juice
   OR 1 Tbsp orange juice
   + 1 Tbsp lime juice
1 Tbsp extra virgin olive oil
3 Tbsp filtered water

1. Blend the achiote and cumin seeds in a coffee or spice grinder. Pour into a small mixing bowl.

2. Stir in the oregano, garlic, allspice, salt and pepper.

3. Add the bitter orange juice, water and enough olive oil to create a thin sauce.

MAKES ½ CUP
4 SERVINGS

Use to marinate 1½ lb chicken, beef or fish. Marinate fish 30 minutes; marinate chicken 1 hour; marinate beef 2-3 hours.

Beta-Carotene • 24mcg
Omega-3 •48mg
Vitamin E • 3%DV

Asian Miso Dressing

1 carrot, roughly chopped
1½ Tbsp fresh ginger,
   roughly minced
1 Tbsp white miso
¼ cup Asian dark vinegar or
   rice vinegar
2 tsp soy sauce or tamari
1 tsp dark sesame oil
1 garlic clove, mashed
¼ tsp black pepper
¼ cup extra virgin olive oil
1 tsp raw honey, optional
½ tsp Sambal, optional
2 Tbsp cilantro, minced

1. Place all ingredients, except the cilantro, into a blender. Puree until smooth.

2. Add cilantro and pulse 2-3 times just to combine.

3. Keep refrigerated for up to 10 days until use.

MAKES 1 CUP • 8 SERVINGS

Beta-Carotene • 653mcg
Omega-3 • 64mg
Vitamin E • 5%DV

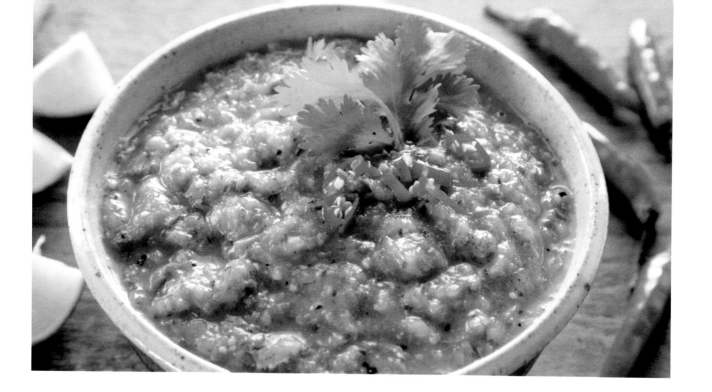

Salsa Verde

1 lb tomatillos,
  husks removed
1 cup sweet onion,
  coarsely chopped
1-2 jalapeños
2 tsp extra virgin olive oil

3 scallions, coarsely
  chopped
1 garlic clove, minced
¼ tsp sea salt
¼ tsp black pepper
¼ cup cilantro, roughly
  chopped

1. Place tomatillos, onion and jalapeños in a heat safe baking dish. Drizzle with olive oil and stir to coat.

2. Preheat broiler to high. Broil until lightly browned, turning 2-3 times. Watch closely to avoid burning.

3. Remove from oven and allow to cool 15 minutes.

4. Pull the stem from the jalapeños. Remove ribs and seeds from jalapeños, if desired.

5. Place the tomatillos, onions, jalapeños, scallions, garlic, salt and pepper into the bowl of a food processor. Puree until smooth. Add the cilantro and pulse 3-4 times.

MAKES 2 CUPS • SERVES 8

Beta-Carotene • 127mcg
Lutein+Zeaxanthin • 391mg
Vitamin C • 18%DV

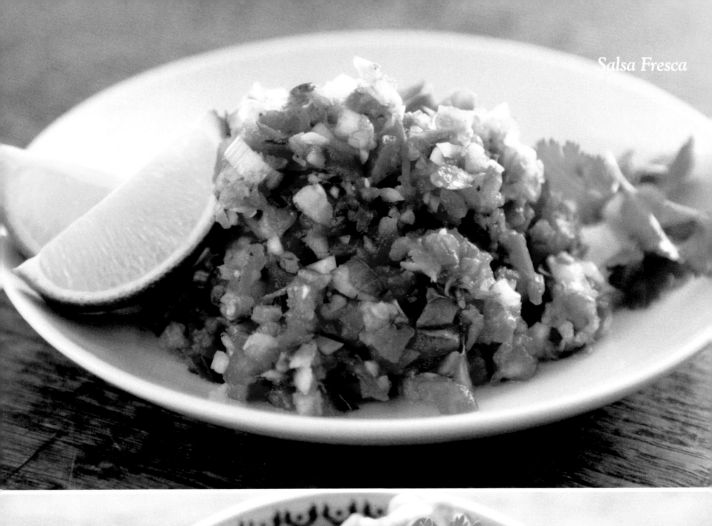

Salsa Fresca

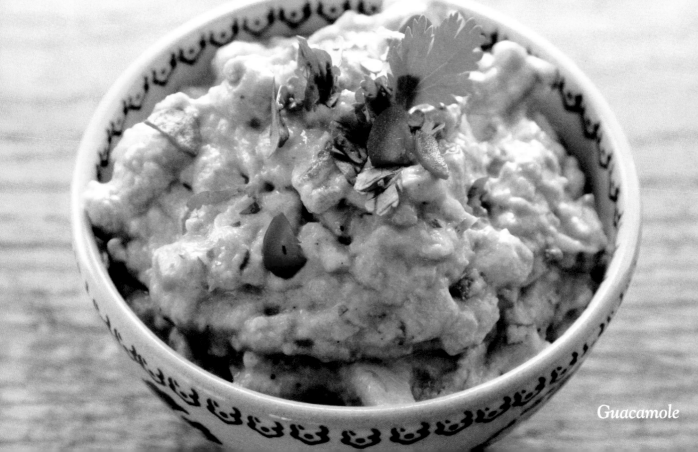

Guacamole

Salsa Fresca

1 lb ripe Roma tomatoes, roughly chopped

½ sweet onion, roughly chopped

1 large garlic clove, finely minced

1 small jalapeño, ribs and seeds removed, finely minced

½ tsp sea salt

¼ tsp black pepper

3 large scallions, diced

½ cup cilantro or Italian flat leaf parsley

1. Place tomatoes, onions, garlic, jalapeño, salt and pepper into the food processor. Pulse 5 or 6 times.

2. Add scallions and cilantro or parsley, pulse 2-3 more times.

3. Serve immediately or refrigerate until ready to use.

MAKES 4 CUPS • SERVES 8

Beta-Carotene • 355mcg
Lycopene • 1,441mcg
Vitamin C • 19%DV

Guacamole

2 avocados, ripe

½ cup scallions, sliced

1 Roma tomato, small dice

3 Tbsp Greek yogurt, non- or low-fat

¼ cup cilantro, minced

1 Tbsp lime juice

1 garlic clove, finely minced

½ tsp hot sauce of choice

¼ tsp sea salt

¼ tsp black pepper

1. In a mixing bowl, mash the avocado with a fork or pastry blender, leaving smooth or chunky as desired.

2. Stir in the remaining ingredients.

3. Garnish with cilantro, chili or jalapeño. Serve immediately or refrigerate until ready to use.

MAKES 1½ CUPS • SERVES 8

Lycopene • 293mcg
Lutein+Zeaxanthin • 191mcg
Vitamin C • 13%DV

Kalamata Lemon Spread

12.3 oz box silken-firm tofu
1 Tbsp mustard, Dijon-style
1 Tbsp lemon juice
¼ tsp lemon zest
1 garlic clove, crushed
¼ tsp sea salt
¼ tsp black pepper
⅓ cup kalamata olives,
   finely minced
¼ cup sun dried tomatoes,
   finely minced
2 Tbsp Italian
   flat leaf parsley

1. Place the tofu, mustard, lemon juice, lemon zest, garlic, salt and pepper into a food processor. Blend until smooth.

2. Add the olives, sun dried tomatoes, and parsley. Pulse 4-5 times until desired consistency is achieved.

MAKES 2 CUPS • 8 SERVINGS

Lycopene • 775mcg
Lutein+Zeaxanthin • 103g
Zinc • 2%DV

Chipotle Garlic Spread

12.3 oz box silken-firm tofu
1-2 chipotle chilies from a
   can of chipotle in adobo
   sauce, minced
1 Tbsp adobo sauce
1 garlic clove, finely minced
1 Tbsp lime juice
½ tsp sea salt
¼ tsp black pepper
3 Tbsp sun dried tomatoes,
   finely minced
3 Tbsp cilantro, minced

1. Place the tofu, chipotle chilies, adobo sauce, garlic, lime juice, salt and pepper into a food processor. Blend until smooth.

2. Add sun dried tomatoes and cilantro. Pulse just to combine.

MAKES 1 ½ CUPS • 6 SERVINGS

Delicious served with steamed artichokes.

Lycopene • 775mcg
Lutein+Zeaxanthin • 44mcg
Zinc • 3%DV

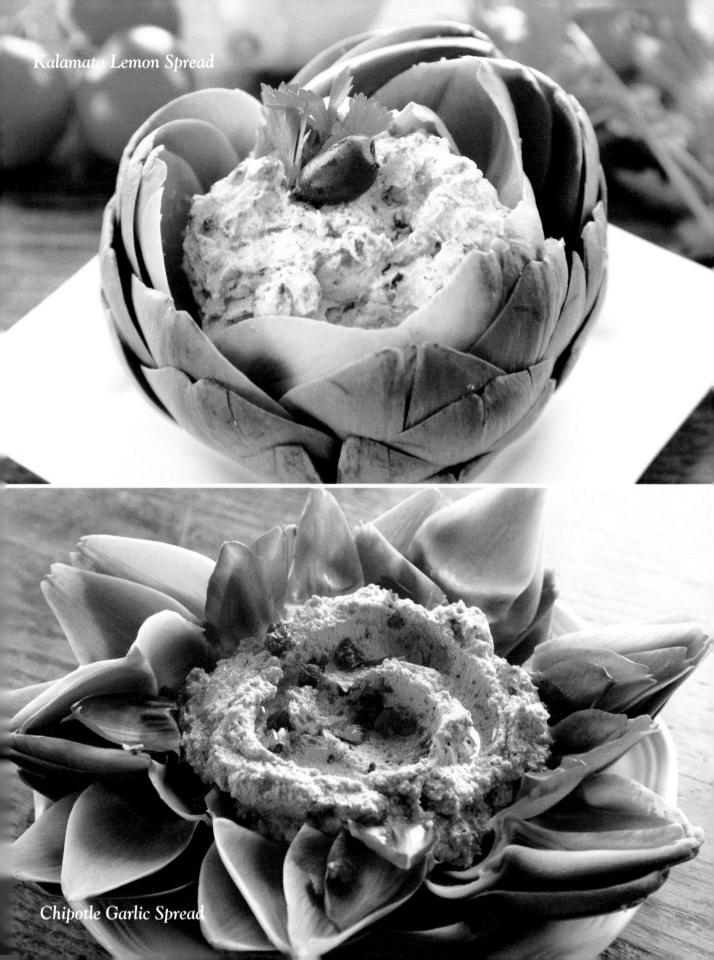

Kalamata Lemon Spread

Chipotle Garlic Spread

Indian Yogurt Marinade

1 cup plain Greek yogurt,
 non- or low-fat
⅓ cup shallot, finely minced
2 garlic cloves, minced
2 tsp fresh ginger, grated
1 Tbsp lime juice

¼ tsp lime zest
½ tsp turmeric
½ tsp paprika,
 smoked or sweet
1 tsp coriander seeds,
 crushed

1 tsp Garam Masala
 (page 202)
½ tsp sea salt
¼ tsp black pepper
1 Tbsp raw honey, optional
1½ tsp hot sauce, optional

1. In a mixing bowl, stir all ingredients together until incorporated.

2. Keep refrigerated for up to 2 days.

MAKES 1¼ CUPS

Use to marinate 1½ lb chicken or beef. Great as a condiment or dip.

Lutein+Zeaxanthin • 35mcg
Vitamin B12 • 6%DV
Zinc • 5%DV

Tzatziki Dip

1 cup cucumbers, quartered
 and finely diced
1¼ cups plain Greek yogurt,
 non- or low-fat
1 large garlic clove, minced
2 tsp fresh dill, chopped
¼ tsp lemon zest
2 tsp lemon juice
1 tsp extra virgin olive oil
⅛ tsp sea salt
⅛ tsp black pepper

Garnish with fresh dill and
 diced cucumber

1. In a mixing bowl combine all ingredients except the garnish. Mix thoroughly.

2. Garnish and serve immediately or refrigerate for up to 3 days.

MAKES 3½ CUPS

Zinc • 3%DV

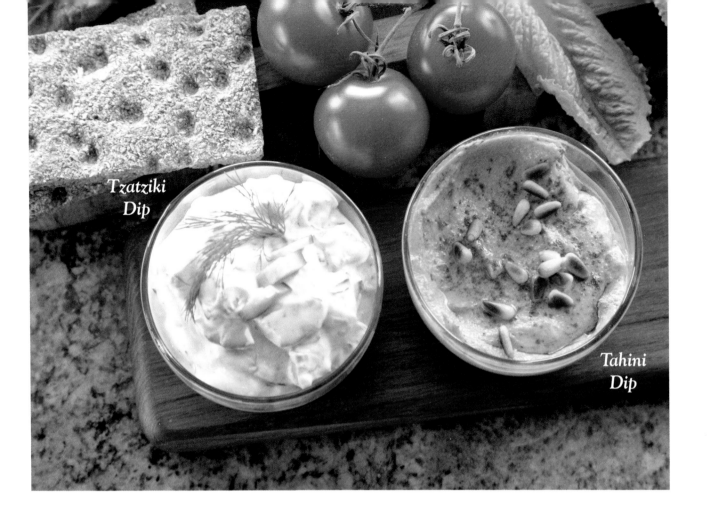

Tzatziki Dip

Tahini Dip

Tahini Dip

½ cup tahini, store-bought
¼ cup lemon juice
¼ cup water
½ tsp garlic powder
½ tsp onion powder
½ tsp smoked paprika
¼ tsp turmeric
½ tsp black pepper
¼ tsp sea salt
1 scallion, diced

½ tsp extra virgin olive oil
1 Tbsp pine nuts, toasted
Pinch of smoked paprika

1. In a mixing bowl, stir together tahini, lemon juice and water until a creamy texture is achieved.

2. Add the remaining spices and scallions. Stir to combine.

3. Place in serving bowl. Garnish with a pinch of smoked paprika and olive oil. Top with toasted pine nuts.

4. Serve immediately or refrigerate for up to 3 days.

MAKES 1 CUP

Lutein+Zeaxanthin • 92mcg
Omega-3 • 63mg
Zinc • 10%DV

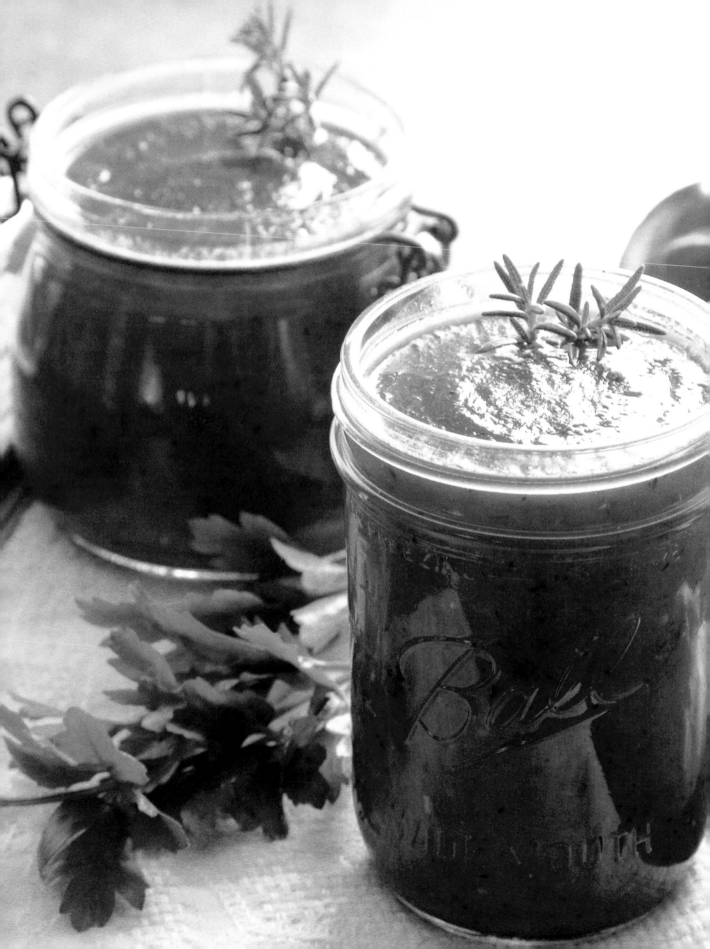

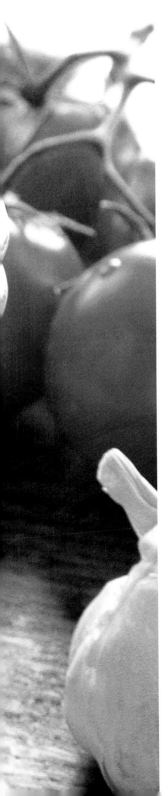

Fresh Marinara

2 Tbsp extra virgin olive oil
1 medium sweet onion, diced
2 garlic cloves, minced
6 oz can tomato paste

1½ lb Roma tomatoes, very ripe, quartered
½ cup filtered water
1 Tbsp Italian seasoning
1 Tbsp dried oregano
1 Tbsp fresh or dried rosemary
¼ tsp black pepper
¼ tsp red pepper flakes
½ tsp sea salt
¼ cup Italian flat leaf parsley, chopped

1. Preheat a large saute pan to medium, add olive oil quickly followed by the onions and garlic. Sauté until softened, 3-4 minutes.

2. Add the tomato paste and sauté 2-3 additional minutes, stirring often. Remove from the heat and set aside.

3. Place the tomatoes and water into a high-speed blender. Puree until smooth.

4. Add the onion mixture to the pureed tomatoes. Puree on high until very smooth. Return to the sauce pan.

5. Add the Italian seasoning, oregano, rosemary, black pepper, red pepper and salt. Simmer for 15-30 minutes.

6. Just before serving, stir in the fresh parsley.

MAKES 5 CUPS • SERVES 10

Lycopene • 5,757mcg
Lutein+Zeaxanthin • 178mcg
Vitamin C • 25%DV

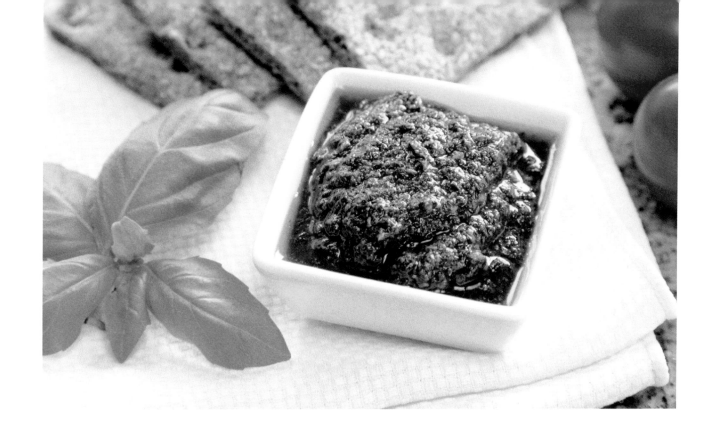

Parsley Basil Pesto

1 ¼ cups Italian flat leaf
   parsley leaves,
   lightly packed
1 ¼ cups basil leaves, cleaned
   and dried, lightly packed
3 garlic cloves, minced

¼ tsp sea salt
¼ tsp black pepper
¼ tsp red pepper flakes
1 Tbsp lemon juice
½ cup extra virgin olive oil

¼ cup Romano or
   Parmesan cheese,
   finely grated
¼ cup walnuts,
   lightly toasted

1. Place parsley, basil, garlic, salt, pepper, red pepper, and lemon juice in the bowl of a food processor.

2. With the food processor running, drizzle in the olive oil stopping occasionally to wipe down the sides.

3. Add the cheese and walnuts. Pulse 5-6 times to combine.

MAKES 1 CUP • SERVES 16

The pesto recipe can be made using a combination of leafy greens and herbs of your choice, such as kale, basil and parsley.

Lutein+Zeaxanthin • 371mcg
Omega-3 • 227mg
Vitamin E • 5%DV

Asian Cucumber Mignonette

¼ cup tarragon vinegar

¼ cup Asian dark vinegar

¼ cup shallot, very finely minced

¼ tsp black pepper

¼ tsp fresh ginger, grated

2 tsp soy sauce or tamari

1 tsp sambal

½ tsp dark sesame oil

¼ cup cucumbers, very finely minced

2 tsp cilantro, very finely minced

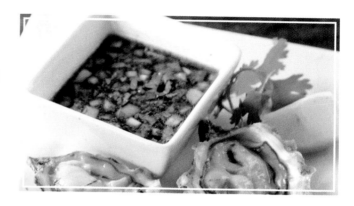

1. Combine all ingredients except the cilantro. If the mignonette is made in advance, add the cilantro just before serving.

2. Keep refrigerated up to 3 days.

MAKES 1 CUP • SERVES 16

Mignonette is a pepper sauce traditionally served with raw oysters. Consider serving the mignonette with steamed clams or mussels.

Beta-Carotene • 12mcg
Lutein+Zeaxanthin • 4mcg
Vitamin C • 2%DV

Cocktail Sauce

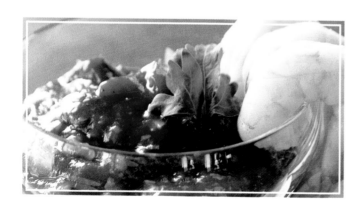

½ cup organic tomato ketchup

2 tsp prepared horseradish

1 Tbsp fresh parsley, minced

1 scallion, finely minced

¼ tsp black pepper

1. Place all ingredients into a mixing bowl. Stir to combine.

2. Keep refrigerated up to 3 days.

MAKES ⅔ CUP • SERVES 3

For an added punch of protein and omega-3's, serve with steamed shrimp or cod.

Lycopene • 4,011mcg
Lutein+Zeaxanthin • 99mcg
Vitamin C • 10%DV

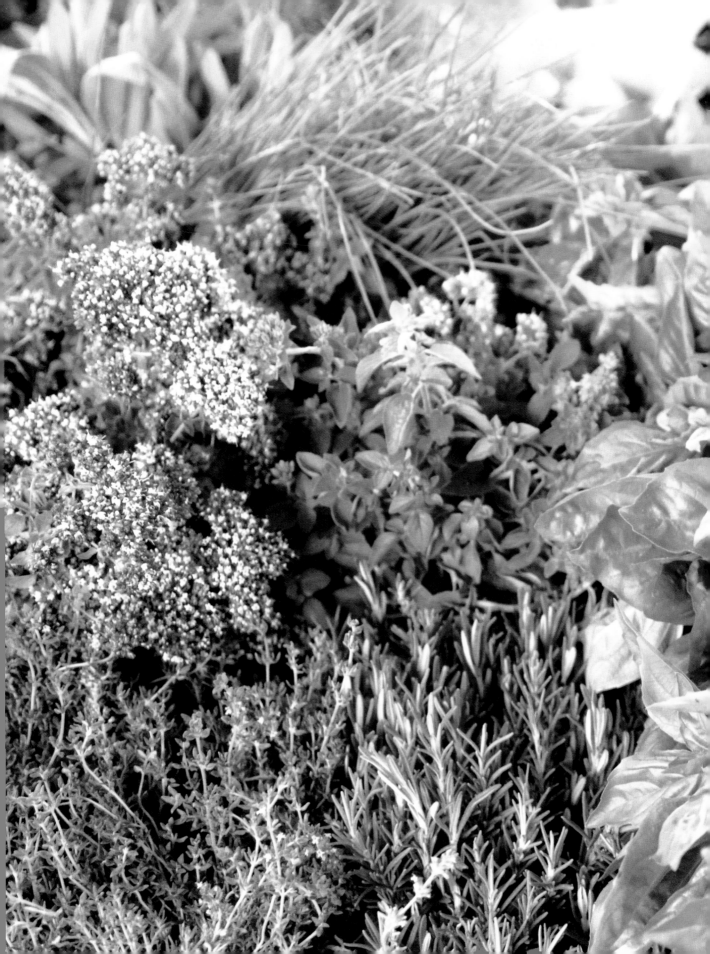

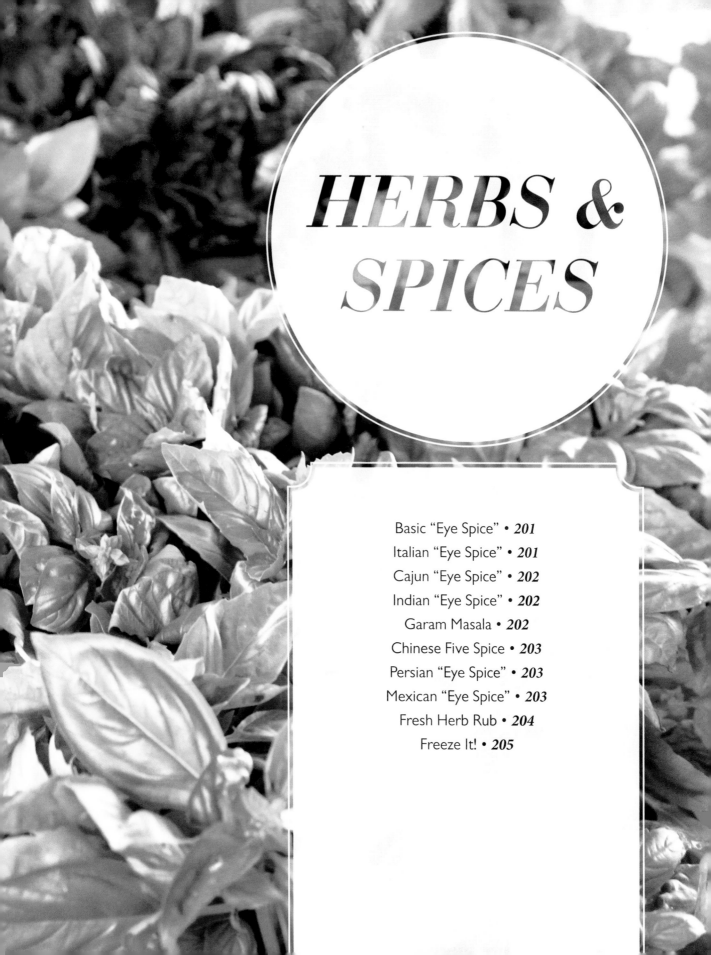

HERBS & SPICES

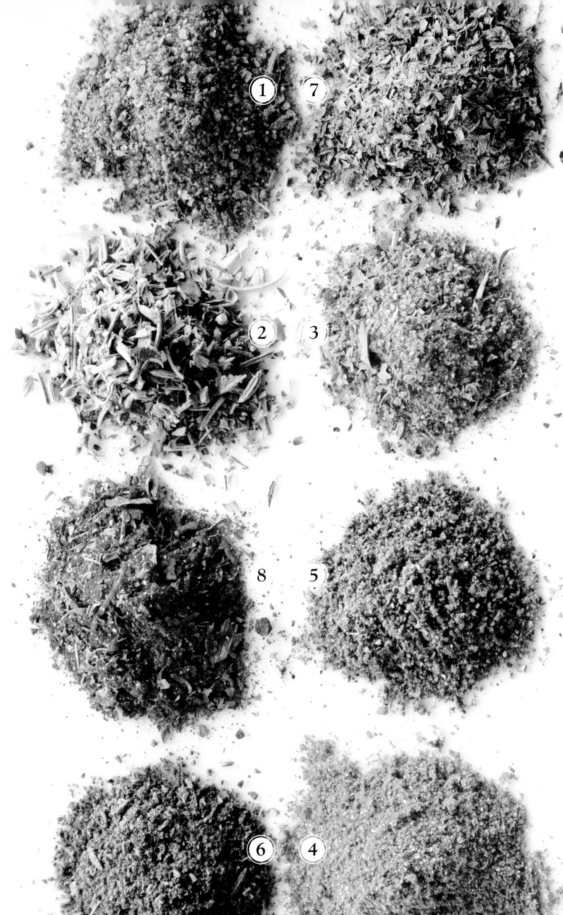

① Basic "Eye Spice"

3 Tbsp dried kale
3 Tbsp ground goji berries
1-½ tsp sea salt, optional
1 Tbsp paprika,
   smoked or sweet
1 Tbsp dried thyme
1 Tbsp dried oregano
1 Tbsp ground ginger
¾ tsp black pepper
2 Tbsp ground sage
1 tsp garlic powder
1 Tbsp dried bouquet garni
2 Tbsp dried parsley
1 tsp onion powder
1 Tbsp ground rosemary
¾ tsp turmeric

1. To make dried kale, use a dehydrator on a low setting or in the oven set to 225°F. Lay kale on a baking sheet or cooling rack and cook until dry and crumbly.

2. While kale is drying, add salt and goji berries to a spice or coffee grinder. Grind until a grainy texture is achieved. Place the goji-salt blend into a mixing bowl. Stir in remaining ingredients.

3. Crumble the dried kale. Stir into the spice blend.

4. Store in a sealed container up to 6 months away from moisture and light.

MAKES 1 CUP

② Italian "Eye Spice"

1 Tbsp parsley
1 Tbsp rubbed sage
1 Tbsp rosemary,
   dried whole leaves
1 Tbsp thyme
1 tsp ground garlic
½ tsp black pepper
1 Tbsp oregano
1 tsp red pepper flakes
1 tsp onion powder
¼ tsp sea salt
1 tsp fennel

1. Combine all ingredients in a small bowl.

2. Store in an airtight container away from moisture and light.

Spice up your favorite tomato sauce. • For a dipping sauce, add spice to balsamic vinegar, fresh chopped parsley and a touch of olive oil. • Sprinkle on halved Roma tomatoes before slow roasting in the oven at 325°F.

MAKES ⅓ CUP

④

Indian "Eye Spice"

2 tsp turmeric
½ tsp garlic powder
½ tsp cumin
½ tsp cinnamon
1 tsp ginger powder
½ tsp cayenne
¼ tsp sea salt
1 tsp coriander seeds
1 tsp black pepper
½ tsp ground cardamom
1 tsp onion powder
3 bay leaves, ground

1. Combine all ingredients in a small bowl.

2. Store in an air tight container away from moisture and light for up to six months.

⑤

Garam Masala

4" cinnamon stick
1 tsp cardamom seeds
2 Tbsp whole cloves
2 Tbsp cumin seeds, whole
1 Tbsp coriander seeds, whole
2 Tbsp black peppercorn, whole

1. Preheat oven to 275°F. Place the spices on a baking sheet. Place into oven and immediately turn **off** the heat. Allow spices to toast for 20 minutes. Remove from the oven and cool to room temperature.

2. Grind all the spices and mix together.

3. Store in an airtight jar for up to 6 months.

③

Cajun "Eye Spice"

3 Tbsp smoked paprika
1 Tbsp oregano
2 tsp thyme
1 tsp onion powder
¼ tsp garlic powder
1 tsp rubbed sage
½ tsp celery seed
3 Tbsp dried parsley
1 tsp cayenne pepper
1 tsp black pepper
½ tsp sea salt

1. Mix all ingredients together.

2. Seal in a jar for up to 6 months.

MAKES ½ CUPS

MAKES ¼ CUP

MAKES ⅔ CUP

Chinese Five Spice

6

4" cinnamon stick, broken into pieces
1 Tbsp whole allspice
4 star anise
1 Tbsp fennel seeds
1 Tbsp Szechuan peppercorns

1. Lightly toast the spices in a dry skillet preheated to medium-low. Stir constantly for 2-3 minutes.

2. Remove from heat to cool to room temperature.

3. Grind in a spice grinder or mortar and pestle.

4. Seal in a jar for up to 6 months.

MAKES ⅓ CUP

Persian "Eye Spice"

7

1½ Tbsp ground cardamom
2 Tbsp cinnamon
1½ Tbsp coriander seeds, crushed
1 Tbsp ground cumin
1 tsp nutmeg
1 tsp powdered ginger
½ tsp ground cloves
½ tsp black pepper
¼ cup dried parsley

1. Combine and store in an airtight jar. Use within 6 months.

A warm, exotic and complex blend of flavors suitable for seasoning lamb and lebneh.

MAKES ⅔ CUPS

Mexican "Eye Spice"

8

2 Tbsp achiote seeds
1 tsp whole black peppercorns
¼ tsp garlic powder
½ tsp ground cumin
2 tsp Mexican oregano
1 tsp turmeric
¼ tsp sea salt

1. Grind achiote and peppercorns in a coffee or spice grinder to a fine powder.

2. Empty contents of the grinder into a small bowl, then add remaining ingredients. Mix to combine.

3. Store in an air tight container away from moisture and light.

MAKES 3 TBSP

Fresh Herb Rub

- 1 Tbsp fresh rosemary, finely chopped
- 2 Tbsp fresh thyme, finely chopped
- 2 Tbsp fresh oregano, finely chopped
- 1 Tbsp fresh marjoram, finely chopped
- 1 Tbsp fresh basil, finely chopped
- 2 Tbsp fresh parsley, finely chopped
- ½ tsp sea salt
- ¼ tsp black pepper
- 1 Tbsp extra virgin olive oil
- 1 Tbsp whole grain mustard

1. Mix all fresh herbs together. Set aside.

2. Combine equal parts olive oil and Dijon-style mustard, 1-2 Tbsp each. Use this mixture to "paint" your protein of choice.

3. Roll the "painted" protein in the fresh herb mixture to coat. Cook as desired: grill, bake or sauté.

MAKES ½ CUP

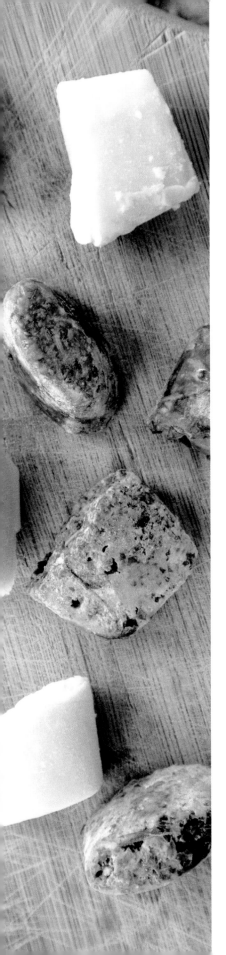

Freeze It!

*A convenient way to use fresh ingredients.
Remove from freezer when ready to use.*

Fresh Herb Ice Cubes

1 cup of freshly chopped herbs, such as:

    oregano
    rosemary
    thyme
    Italian flat leaf parsley
    cilantro
    parsley
    mixed herbs

1. Pick one or more of your favorite herbs listed above.

2. Finely chop the fresh herbs.

3. Place 1 Tbsp chopped herbs into each ice cube mold. Add water to cover.

4. Freeze overnight. Remove and place in an air-tight freezer bag until ready to use.

Coconut Milk Ice Cubes

14.5 oz can coconut milk, light or regular

1. Pour leftover coconut milk into an ice cube tray. Freeze overnight.

2. Remove and seal in an airtight freezer bag.

Pesto Ice Cubes

1 cup Parsley Basil Pesto (page 196)

1. Add 1 Tbsp pesto to ice cube tray. Freeze overnight.

2. Remove and seal in an airtight freezer bag.

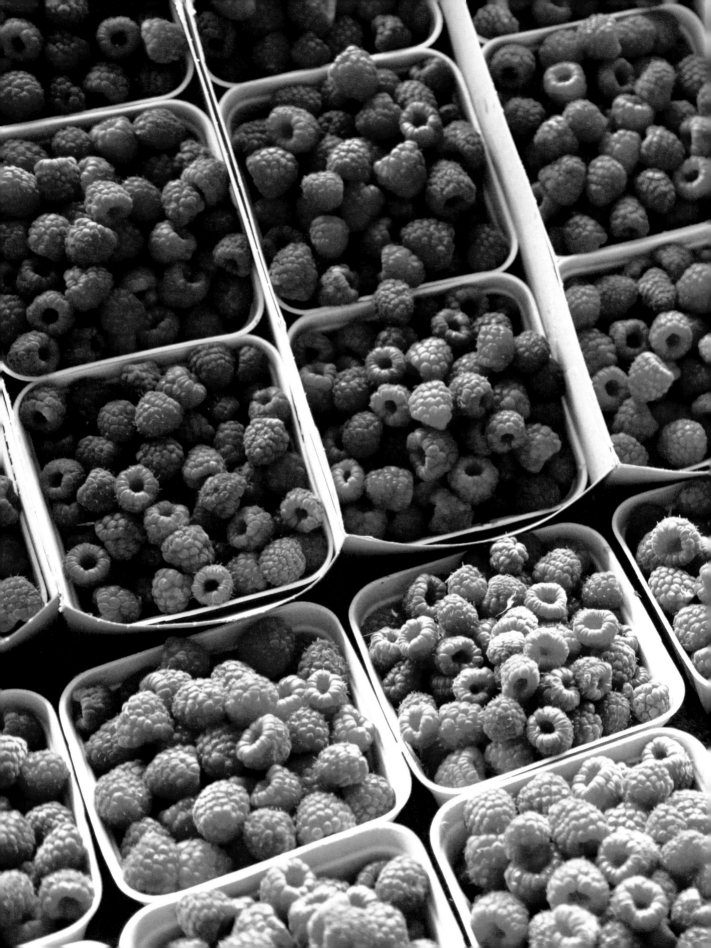

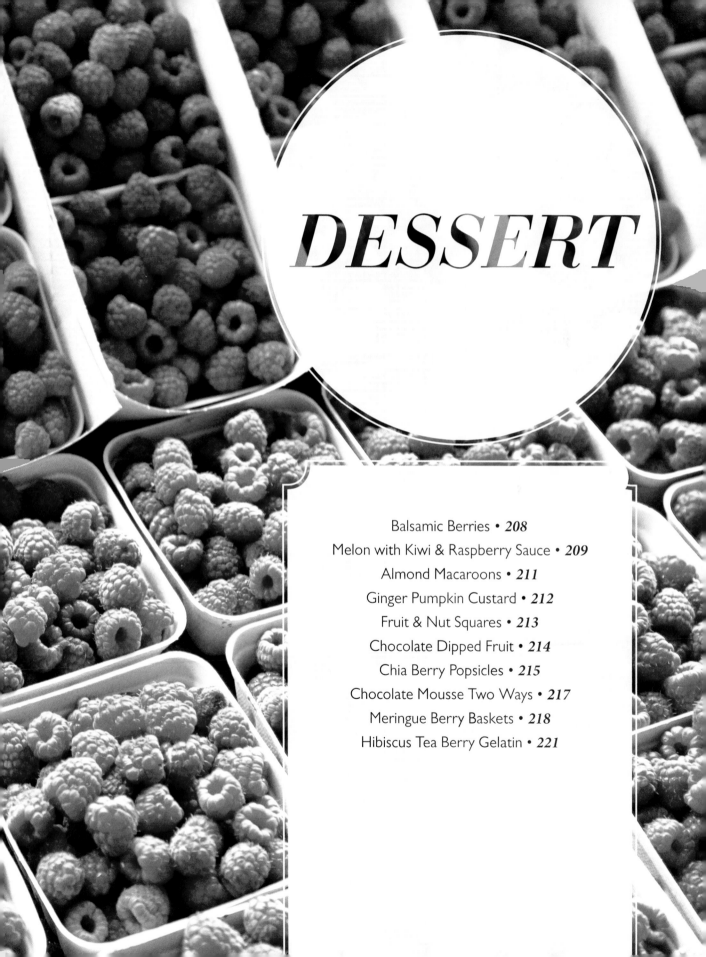

DESSERT

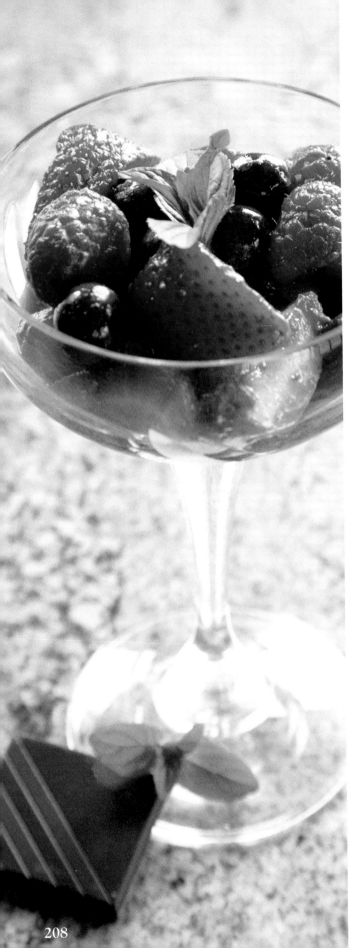

Balsamic Berries

2 cup strawberries, divided
⅛ tsp black pepper
¼ cup balsamic vinegar
1 cup blueberries
1 cup raspberries
1 cup strawberries, quartered
2 Tbsp maple syrup

1. Slice and mash 1 cup strawberries. Quarter the remaining 1 cup.

2. In a mixing bowl, combine mashed strawberries, pepper and balsamic vinegar.

3. Stir in the blueberries, raspberries, quartered strawberries and maple syrup. Allow to macerate for 10-20 minutes.

4. Serve within 1 hour with a wedge of extra-dark chocolate.

SERVES 4

Omega-3 • 110mg
Vitamin C • 94%DV
Zinc • 5%DV

Melon with Kiwi & Raspberry Sauce

for the kiwi sauce
  6 kiwis, peeled

for the raspberry sauce
  12 oz frozen raspberries, thawed

fresh fruit
  2 kiwis, sliced
  ½ honeydew melon, sliced
  I mango, sliced
  ½ pint fresh raspberries
  ½ pint fresh blueberries
  Fresh mint, for garnish

1. To make the kiwi sauce, puree kiwis in the blender until smooth.

2. To make the raspberry sauce, puree the thawed raspberries until smooth. If the raspberries are too tart, add honey to sweeten, to taste.

3. To plate the dessert, arrange the fruit and sauces creatively. This can be done at the table for a fun, entertaining dessert.

SERVES 8

Lutein+Zeaxanthin • 226mcg
Vitamin C • 207%DV
Vitamin E • 11%DV

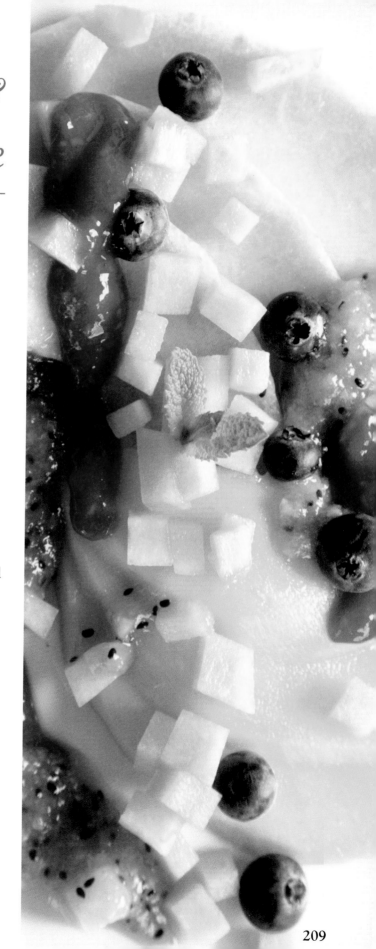

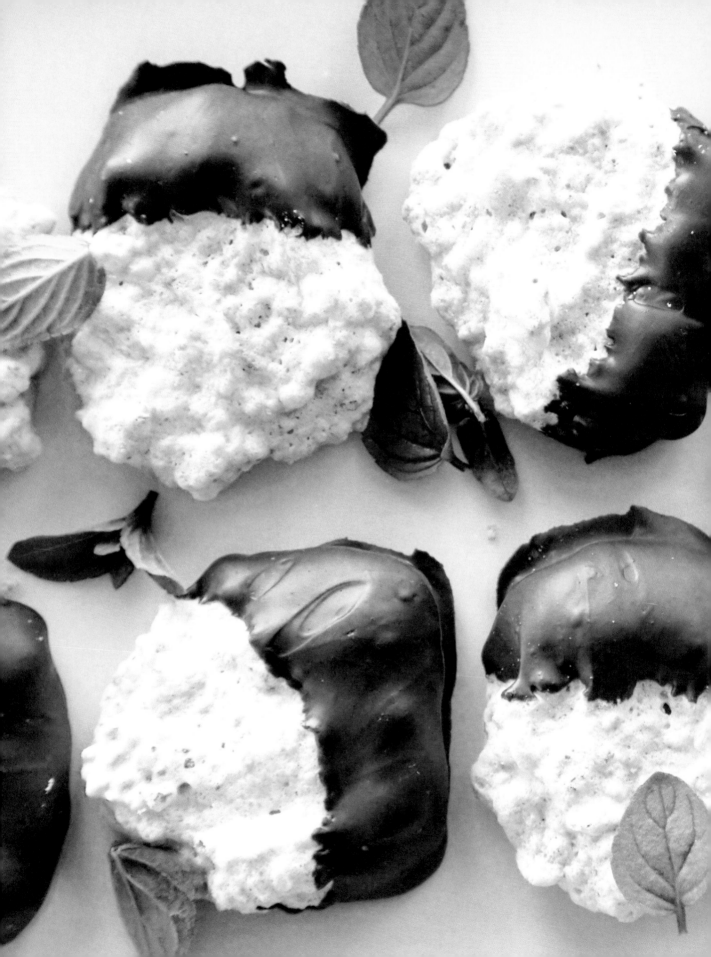

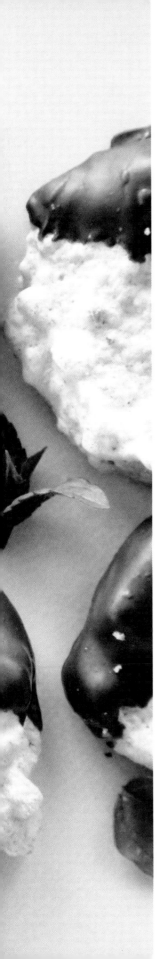

Almond Macaroons

1 ½ cups lightly roasted almonds, ground to a rustic flour

½ cup evaporated cane sugar, divided

3 egg whites, room temperature

Pinch of sea salt

¼ tsp cream of tartar

½ tsp almond extract

½ tsp vanilla extract

6 oz high-quality dark chocolate

2 tsp coconut oil

to lightly roast almonds

Preheat oven to 300°F. Place whole almonds in a single layer on a baking sheet. Bake for 10 minutes. Remove the almonds from the oven to stir. Return the almonds to the oven. Turn oven **off** and leave almonds in the oven with the door closed for 30 minutes.

1. Preheat oven to 300°F. In a mixing bowl, combine almond flour and 2 Tbsp sugar. Set aside.

2. Using an electric mixer, beat egg whites and salt on medium-low until frothy, then add the cream of tartar. Beat until the egg whites form soft peaks. Gradually add the sugar, almond extract and vanilla extract. Beat until shiny stiff peaks are formed.

3. Gently fold the egg whites into the almond flour mixture until well combined.

4. Spoon 2 Tbsp mounds onto parchment lined baking sheets, leaving 1" between cookies.

5. Bake 25-30 minutes, or until edges are light golden. Remove from the oven and allow to rest 2-3 minutes. Transfer to a cooling rack to completely cool.

6. Melt chocolate and coconut oil in the microwave or a double boiler. Spread the bottom of each macaroon with 1 tsp melted chocolate. Place on parchment paper and allow chocolate to harden.

MAKES 30 MACAROONS

Vitamin E • 24%DV
Zinc • 7%DV

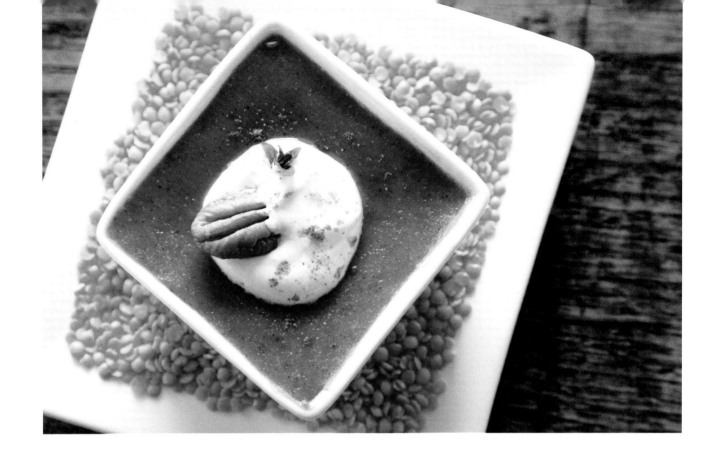

Ginger Pumpkin Custard

15 oz can pumpkin puree
14.5 can light coconut milk
2 omega-3 eggs
1 Tbsp molasses
⅓ cup raw honey
2 tsp cinnamon
1¼ tsp fresh ginger, grated
   or ¾ tsp dried ginger
¼ tsp ground cloves
¼ tsp ground allspice
¼ tsp white pepper
¼ tsp sea salt

1. Preheat oven to 350°F. Place all ingredients in a mixing bowl. Whisk very well to combine.

2. Pour into a lightly greased 1½ qt baking dish. Bake for 50-60 minutes. The custard will be done when the center has set and a knife comes out clean when inserted halfway between the center and the edge.

MAKES 4 CUPS • SERVES 8

Consider serving with coconut whipped cream (page 217).

Omega-3 • 106mg
Folate • 6%DV
Zinc • 15%DV

Fruit & Nut Squares

1 cup dried Pacific apricots
½ cup medjool dates, pitted
½ cup dried cherries
½ cup lightly roasted walnuts
  (see directions below)
2 Tbsp orange juice
Zest of 1 orange
½ cup unsweetened
  shredded coconut

**to lightly roast pecans
and walnuts**

Preheat oven to 300°F.
Place pecans or walnuts in
a single layer on a baking
sheet. Place in the oven and
turn **off** the heat. Allow to
roast for 30 minutes.

1. Add the apricots, dates, cherries and walnuts to the
bowl of a food processor. Process until finely chopped.
Add the orange juice and zest; pulse 2-3 times to
combine.

2. Drop 2 tsp size spoonfuls into the coconut shreds.
Using your hands, shape into cubes.

3. Store in an airtight container for up to 4 weeks.

MAKES 30 SQUARES • SERVES 15

Beta-Carotene • 204mcg
Omega-3 • 359mg
Vitamin E • 2%DV

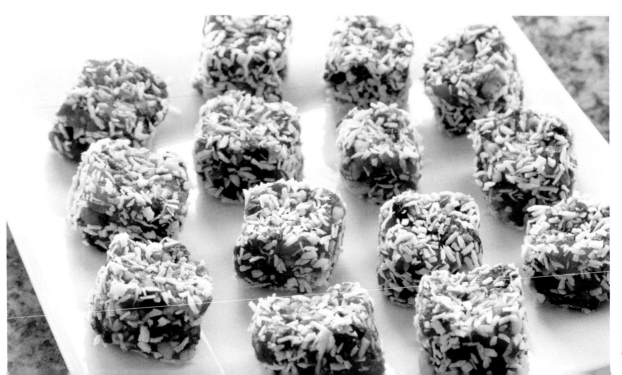

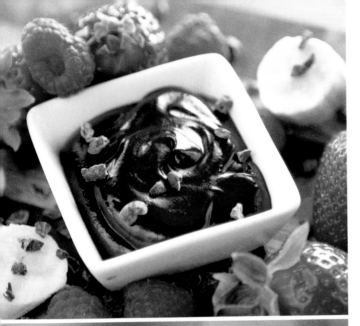

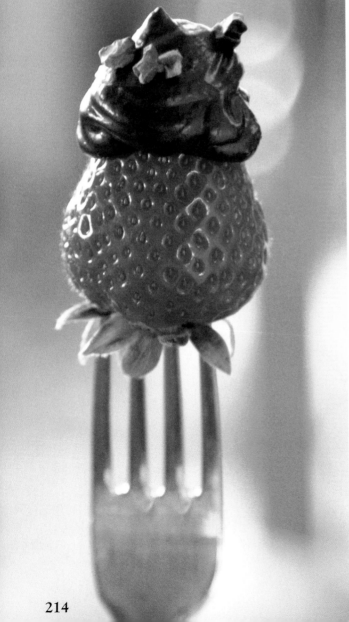

Chocolate Dipped Fruit

4 oz unsweetened chocolate	1 Tbsp agave nectar
	¼ tsp vanilla extract
2 Tbsp coconut oil	⅛ tsp sea salt

5 Tbsp maple syrup, grade B	1 Tbsp cacao nibs
	20 strawberries
3 Tbsp unsweetened soymilk	20 raspberries
2 tsp instant coffee granules	4 bananas, cut into bite-sized chunks

1. In a heat safe bowl, microwave chocolate and coconut oil on high in 30 second intervals. Stir and repeat until completely melted. Set aside.

2. Combine maple syrup and soy milk. Microwave on high until very hot. Stir in coffee to dissolve, then the agave, vanilla and salt.

3. Whisk melted chocolate into the coffee mixture until smooth and shiny.

4. Transfer into a serving bowl, sprinkle with cacao nibs and serve with fresh fruit, such as strawberries, raspberries and bananas.

MAKES 1 CUP • SERVES 8

Vitamin B6 • 12%DV
Vitamin C • 40%DV
Zinc • 14%DV

Chia Berry Popsicles

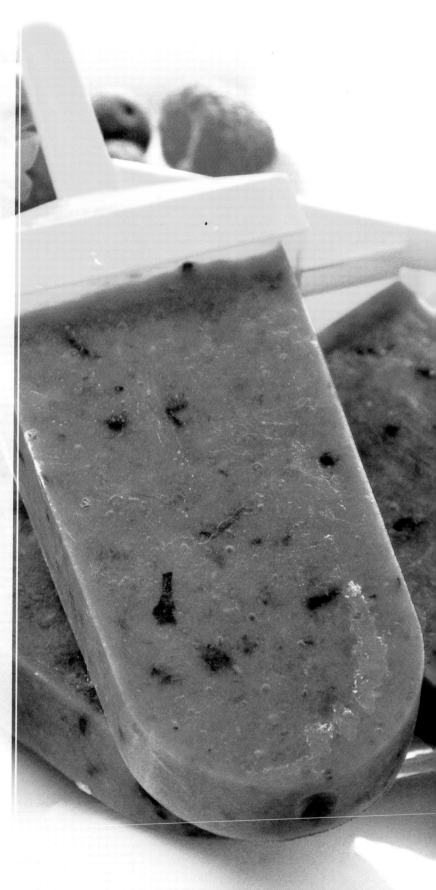

3 Tbsp chia seeds
+ ½ cup water

1¾ cup fresh or frozen
mixed berries

1 kiwi, peeled

⅓ cup plain Greek yogurt,
non- or low-fat

1 Tbsp lemon juice

⅓ cup açaí juice

1. Stir chia seeds into the water. Let this mixture sit for 15 minutes to hydrate the chia seeds.

2. Place all ingredients, including the chia mixture, into a blender. Blend until smooth or chunky as desired.

3. Pour into a popsicle mold or create your own mold with juice glasses and wooden popsicle sticks.

4. Freeze until ready to enjoy.

MAKES 8 POPSICLES

Lutein+Zeaxanthin • 41mcg
Omega-3 • 885mg
Vitamin C • 32%DV

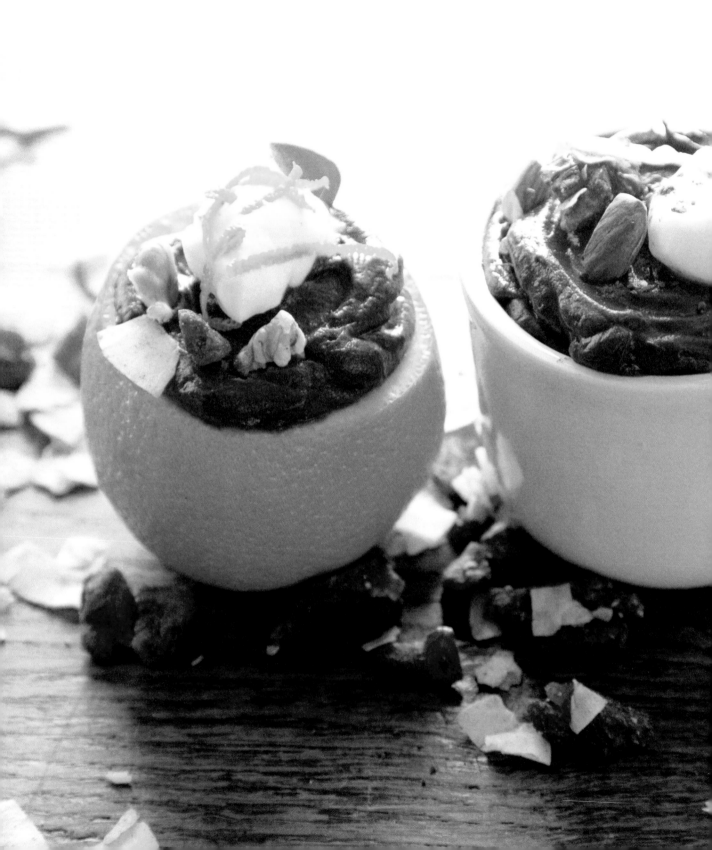

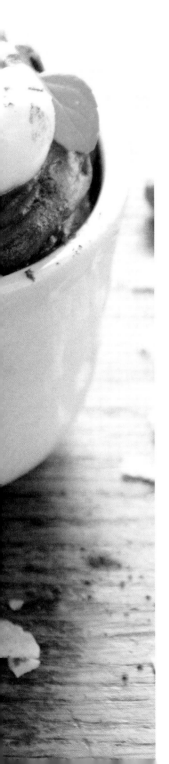

**almond
chocolate mousse**

2 large ripe avocados
⅓ cup natural cocoa powder
¼ cup agave nectar
2 tsp vanilla extract
1 tsp almond extract
1 tsp açaí powder, optional
Pinch of sea salt

**orange
chocolate mousse**

2 large ripe avocados
⅓ cup natural cocoa powder
¼ cup agave nectar
1 tsp vanilla extract
1 Tbsp orange juice or
 orange liquor
½ tsp orange zest
¼ tsp cinnamon
2 tsp açaí powder, optional
Pinch of sea salt

coconut whipped cream

½ cup full-fat coconut milk,
 refrigerated overnight
1 Tbsp agave nectar,
 optional

for the topping

2 dates, finely diced
¼ cup walnuts
 or almonds, chopped
 Tbsp dehydrated
2 shredded coconut flakes,
 toasted

1. Combine the topping ingredients in a small bowl. Stir to combine and set aside.

2. Place all ingredients for either the almond or orange mousse into a food processor and process until completely smooth. This mixture can be made ahead. Keep refrigerated.

3. Without shaking, open the can of coconut milk and scoop the cream off the top. Whip with an electric mixer. Add the agave nectar. Use the coconut milk remaining the in the can 1 Tbsp at a time as needed to achieve a light, fluffy whipped cream.

4. To serve, portion the mousse, topping and whipped cream into small cups.

SERVES 6

ALMOND CHOCOLATE MOUSSE

Lutein+Zeaxanthin • 128mcg
Vitamin E • 12%DV
Zinc • 13%DV

ORANGE CHOCOLATE MOUSSE

Lutein+Zeaxanthin • 127mcg
Omega-3 • 493mg
Zinc • 11%DV

Meringue Berry Baskets

4 egg whites,
   room temperature
Pinch of sea salt
¼ tsp cream of tarter
½ cup evaporated
   cane sugar
1 tsp vanilla extract

1 recipe Chia Berry Sauce
   (page 38)
3 cups fresh berries

Fresh mint, to garnish

1. Preheat oven to 225°F. Using an electric mixer, beat egg whites and salt on medium speed until frothy. Add the cream of tarter. Beat until soft peaks have formed.

2. Gradually add sugar 1 Tbsp at a time, until stiff peaks have formed. Beat in the vanilla extract.

3. Line 2 baking sheets with parchment paper. Transfer egg whites to a pastry bag fitted with a star tip. To create baskets, pipe 10-3" diameter circles. Fill in circles with meringue. Pipe a second layer of stars to the perimeter. Alternatively, use a large spoon to create simple cloud-like mounds.

4. Bake for 1½ hours. Turn the heat off and cool in the oven for an additional 2-3 hours, leaving the door closed.

5. To assemble, place 1 meringue onto each dessert plate. Add 2 Tbsp chia sauce to the meringue basket. Garnish with fresh berries and a sprig of mint. The meringue baskets would also be delicious served with Balsamic Berries (page 208).

SERVES 10

Omega-3 • 398mg
Vitamin C • 43%DV
Zinc • 12%DV

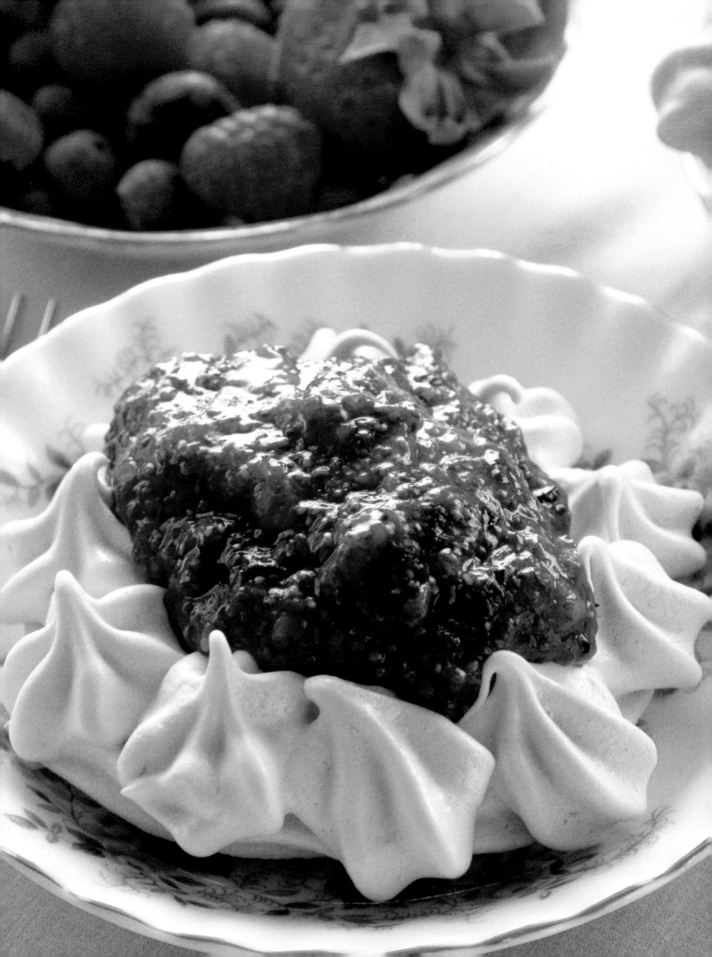

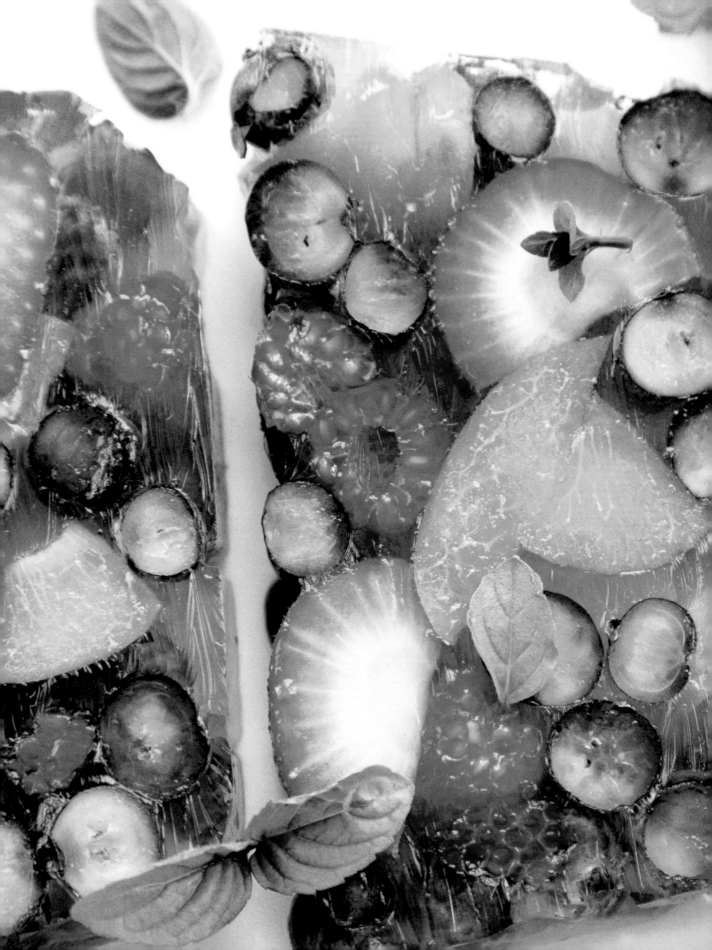

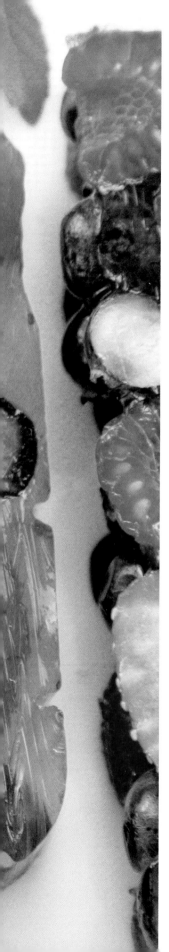

Hibiscus Tea Berry Gelatin

3 packages dried unflavored gelatin

3¼ cups water

½ cup evaporated cane sugar

2 Tbsp dried hibiscus flowers, also known as "flor de Jamaica"

1 tsp rosewater

6 cups fresh berries and fruit, such as blueberries, strawberries, raspberries, peaches and apricots

Do not use kiwi, pineapple or papaya as they interfere with gelatin's ability to set.

1. Add the dried gelatin to 1 cup cold water. Allow to sit.

2. Bring 2¼ cups water to a boil. Add sugar and hibiscus flowers. Remove from the heat and allow to steep for 15 minutes. Pour through strainer into a mixing bowl.

3. Add the rose water and soaked gelatin to the hibiscus tea. Stir until the gelatin has completely dissolved. Add the berries and pour into a 4"×8" glass loaf pan.

4. Refrigerate 3-4 hours or overnight until set. To unmold, place loaf pan in hot water for 30 seconds. Slice and serve.

6 SERVINGS

Lutein+Zeaxanthin • 97mcg
Omega-3 • 71mg
Vitamin C • 53%DV

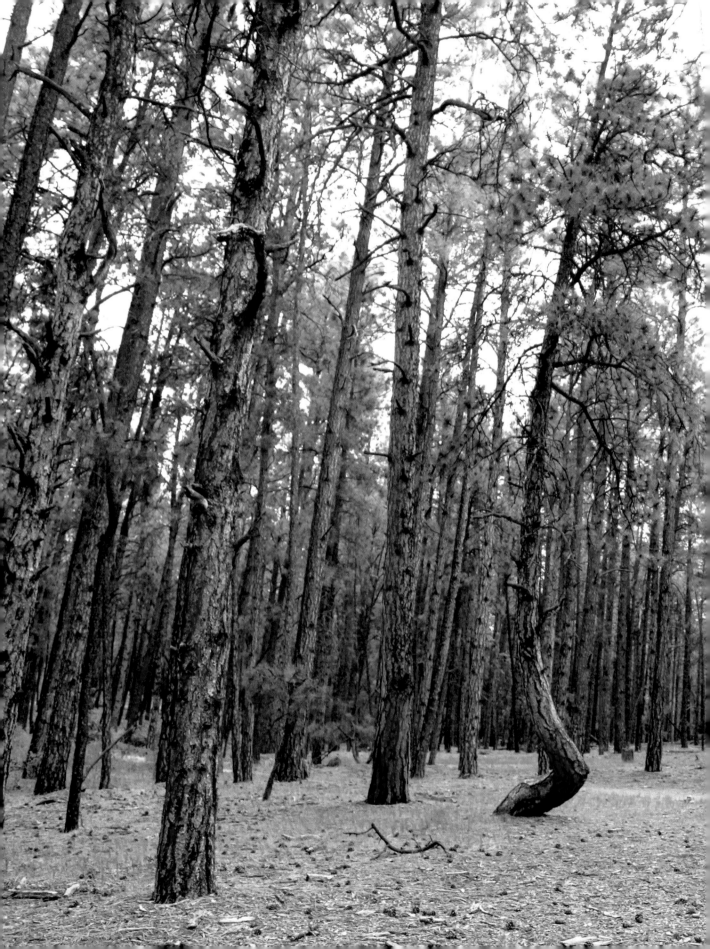

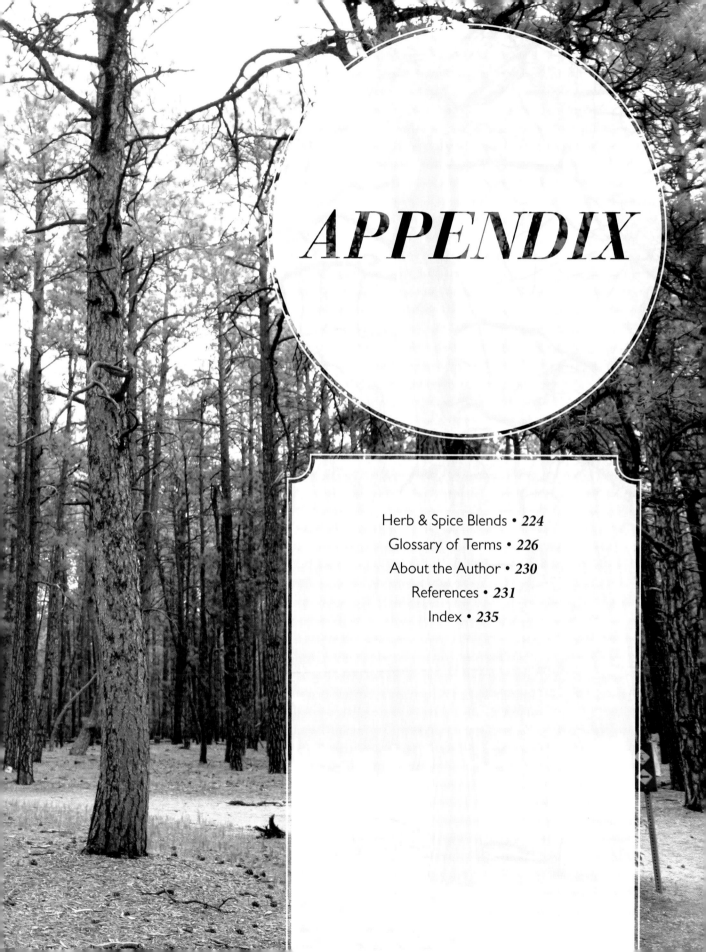

APPENDIX

Herb & Spice Blends

Organic herbs and spices are nutritionally potent "supplements" from the garden. The following is a collection of herb and spice blends to enhance the flavor and health benefits of your meals.

herb/spice	nutritional attributes	tasty combinations
Basil	Vitamins A, C, K; Fiber, Omega-3, Zinc, Beta-Carotene, Lutein+Zeaxanthin, Orientin, Vicenin, Eugenol	+ garlic, oregano, rosemary, parsley + scallions, garlic, ginger, red pepper flakes, turmeric, fish sauce + cumin, mexican oregano, cilantro, jalapeño
Bay Leaf	Vitamins A, B6; Iron, Manganese, Cineol	+ parsley, thyme, peppercorn, marjoram, onion, chili powder, oregano, celery
Parsley	Vitamins A, C, K; Beta-Carotene, Lutein+Zeaxathin, Apigenin	+ garlic, lemon zest and juice, capers, black pepper + thyme, bay leaf, dill, tarragon, chives + paprika, cumin, fennel, black pepper + sage, rosemary, thyme, garlic, magoram
Turmeric	Vitamin B6, Manganese, Iron, Curcumin	+ chili pepper, coriander, cumin, mustard seeds, curry leaves, ginger, black peppercorn + ginger, cumin, coriander, paprika, cayenne + garlic, ginger, coconut, onion, saffron
Cinnamon	Dietary Fiber, Manganese, Calcium, Iron, Cinnamaldehyde	+ nutmeg, cloves, allspice, white pepper + cardamom, cloves, ginger, orange zest, black pepper, coriander, turmeric
Cayenne, Red Pepper Flakes, Paprika	Vitamins A, C, B6; Beta-Carotene, Lutein+Zeaxanthin, Capsaicin	+ chili powder, onion powder, cilantro, cumin, garlic + thyme, oregano, black pepper, onion powder, marjoram, rosemary, fennel seed
Black Pepper	Vitamin K, Manganese, Dietary Fiber, Iron, Piperine	+ everything! salads, vegetables, entrées + lemon zest and juice, garlic, parsley, dill + cardamom, cinnamon, coconut milk, cloves, star anise
Ginger	Dietary Fiber, Vitamin B6, Copper, Manganese, Gingerol	+ garlic, soy sauce, cilantro, wasabi, sesame oil, scallions + cinnamon, allspice, nutmeg, white pepper, cloves + mango, lime, cilantro, jalapeño
Dill	Vitamin A, Calcium, Iron, Kaempferol, Vicenin	+ mint, garlic, bay leaf, parsley, lemon + horseradish, parsley, capers, garlic, black pepper + lemon, scallions, garlic, parsley
Cilantro	Vitamins K, A; Beta-Carotene, Lutein+Zeaxanthin, Quercitin, Kaempferol, Apigenin, Rhamnetin	+ red onion, garlic, cumin, Mexican oregano, black pepper, ground achiote seeds + ginger, garlic, wasabi, sesame oil, red pepper flakes, scallions
Rosemary	Dietary Fiber, Calcium, Iron, Carnosol, Rosmanol, Rosmarinic Acid	+ parsley, sage, oregano, thyme, garlic, red pepper flakes + marjoram, oregano, thyme, garlic, dill, parsley, basil + mint, garlic, cumin, basil, thyme, lemon zest
Onion, Green Onion, Chives	Dietary Fiber, Vitamins B6, C; Chromium, Quercitin	+ oregano, black pepper, garlic + marjoram, parsley, sage, rosemary + smoked paprika, garlic, black pepper, parsley

herb/spice	nutritional attributes	tasty combinations
Shallot	Vitamins A, B6, C, K; Folate, Iron, Copper, Manganese, Zinc, Beta-Carotene, Lutein+Zeaxanthin, Quercetin, Kaempferol, Sulpher-Containing Antioxidant Compounds	+ garlic, thyme, rosemary, orange zest, parsley, cloves, red wine + mint, dill, parsley, marjoram + ginger, garlic, lime, cilantro, red pepper flakes
Anise Seed	Vitamins B6, C, Iron, Zinc, Manganese	+ almond and vanilla extracts, black pepper, cloves, coriander + dried chilies, pepita seeds, cloves, ground achiote seeds, cinnamon, Mexican chocolate
Cumin	Iron, Manganese, Beta-Carotene, Lutein+Zeaxanthin, Cuminaldehyde	+ turmeric, cilantro, bay leaf, cinnamon, cloves, cardamom, black pepper + garlic, ginger, garam masala, turmeric, cilantro + garlic, lemon zest, cinnamon, cloves, jalapeño
Thyme	Vitamins A, C, K; Manganese, Lutein+Zeaxanthin, Beta-Carotene, Iron, Thymol	+ cayenne, paprika, garlic, onion powder, black pepper, oregano + onion powder, allspice, cinnamon, paprika, cumin, nutmeg, garlic and black pepper + basil, oregano, rosemary, parsley, red pepper flakes, black pepper
Saffron	Vitamin C, Manganese, Iron, Zeaxanthin, Alpha-Crocin, Safranal	+ shallots, black pepper, parsley, garlic + paprika, rosemary, garlic, oregano, lemon zest
Cardamom	Manganese, Iron, Zinc	+ turmeric, cloves, ginger, anise, mustard, saffron, garlic + orange zest, cinnamon, white pepper
Achiote Seeds	Vitamin E as Tocotrienols, Lycopene, Zeaxanthin, Bixin	+ allspice, chili, citrus juice, cloves, cumin, garlic, Mexican oregano, paprika, pepita seeds
Mustard Seeds	Selenium, Tryptophan, Omega-3, Zinc, Vitamin B3, Lutein+Zeaxanthin, Glucosinolates	+ vinegar, turmeric, tarragon, coriander, cumin + dill, fennel, fenugreek, garlic, honey
Cloves	Lutein+Zeaxanthin, Eugenol	+ cinnamon, fennel, star anise, Szechuan pepper + allspice, cardamom, ginger, mace, nutmeg, white pepper + cardamom, cinnamon, cumin seeds, coriander seeds, bay leaf, black pepper
Oregano	Dietary Fiber, Vitamins B6, A, E, K; Folate, Iron, Manganese, Beta-Carotene, Lutein+Zeaxanthin, Thymol	+ parsley, garlic, capers, lemon zest, thyme, marjoram, black pepper, red pepper flakes + basil, garlic, onion powder, mustard
Marjoram	Vitamins A, K; Folate, Calcium, Iron (Very High), Manganese, Beta-Carotene, Lutein+Zeaxanthin, Eugenol	+ parsley, bay leaf, rosemary, garlic, black pepper + fennel, mustard, orange zest + basil, oregano, thyme, rosemary, sage
Sage	Vitamin K, Beta-Carotene, Lutein+Zeaxanthin, Apgenin, Diosmetin, Rosmarinic Acid	+ thyme, garlic, parsley, basil, oregano, black pepper + fennel seeds, dried ginger, marjoram
Fennel	Dietary Fiber, Calcium, Copper, Iron, Manganese, Kaempferol, Quercetin	+ chervil, thyme, dill, parsley + cloves, cinnamon, star anise, Szechuan pepper
Nutmeg	Dietary Fiber, Copper, Manganese, Cryptoxanthin	+ coriander seeds, cumin seeds, cloves, black pepper, garam masala, cinnamon, cardamom, turmeric + cumin, sweet paprika, bay leaf, turmeric, garlic, black pepper + allspice, cinnamon, ginger, cloves, white pepper

Glossary of Terms

Açaí Berries: Native to South American rainforest, açaí berries are the fruit from the açaí palm tree. They can be purchased as juice or freeze dried and powdered.

Agave nectar: An amber colored, filtered syrup from an agave cactus. Agave is sweeter than honey and has a high-fructose content. Use sparingly.

ALA (alpha-linolenic acid): An essential, polyunsaturated, omega-3 fatty acid from plant sources. Food sources include chia seeds, flax seeds, lingonberry seeds and walnuts.

Achiote (Annatto) Seeds: Grown in tropical and subtropical regions. Annatto seeds are commonly used in Caribbean and Latin cuisine. These seeds are a good source of carotenoids and tocotrioenols (Vitamin E) and can be purchased as dried seeds or as a paste.

Antioxidant: Micronutrients which inhibit a chemical reaction called oxidation. Oxidation can produce free-radicals which can damage cells. Vitamins C and E are examples of antioxidants.

Arrowroot: A gluten-free starch used as a thickener. This starch, thickens to a clear gel at a lower temperatures and should not be overheated.

Asian Dark Vinegar: A rich, malty, dark-colored, rice-based vinegar. Available in Asian supermarkets.

Beta-carotene: An anti-oxidant in a pro-vitamin form of Vitamin A. Beta-carotene is in the carotenoid family. Dietary examples include carrot juice, spinach and sweet potato.

Bioavailability: The extent to which nutrients can be absorbed by cells in the body.

Bioflavonoids (flavonoids): A group of biologically active compounds found in plants, essential for the stability and absorption of Vitamin C. Food sources include berries, green tea, yellow onions and parsley.

Blood glucose: The blood sugar concentration present in the blood.

Bouquet Garni: A fresh herb bundle frequently consisting of savory, rosemary, thyme, oregano, basil, dill, marjoram, sage, tarragon, bay leaf, parsley and/or peppercorns. For the recipes in this book, a dried herb version is used. It can be found in supermarkets and spice stores.

Cacao nibs: Broken pieces of dried, roasted, cocoa beans containing high amounts of theobromine and flavonoids. Cacao nibs can be ground and used in savory dishes, smoothies or as a snack.

Carotenoids: A group of brightly colored pigments synthesized by plants, some of which have antioxidant activity. Food sources include pumpkin, and tomato paste.

Cataracts: An eye condition characterized by a clouding of the normally clear crystalline lens inside of the eye. Cataracts can lead to impairment of vision and are usually treated with surgery.

Chia seeds: Seeds from flowering plants in the mint family, native to Mexico and South America. Chia seeds are rich in ALA omega-3 fatty acids, protein and dietary fiber.

Choroid: A pigmented, vascular layer in the posterior portion of the eye. It lies between the retina and the sclera and provides oxygen and nourishment to the highly metabolic retina. The pigment helps to minimize light scattering within the eye.

Ciliary body: A circular structure located at the base of the iris which is responsible for fluid production and generating accommodation.

Complex carbohydrate: A category of carbohydrate made of oligosaccharides and polysaccharides, rich in fiber, vitamins and minerals. Food sources include broccoli, lentils and whole grains.

Cornea: The transparent, convex, anterior covering of the eye. The cornea transitions to the white (sclera) portion of the eye. The cornea transmits and helps focus light into the eye.

Daily Value (DV): Recommended intake of a nutrient based on a 2,000-2,500 calorie diet.

DHA (Docosahexaenoic acid): An essential, long-chain, polyunsaturated, omega-3 fatty acid. Food sources include herring, salmon, sardines and omega-3 enriched eggs.

Dietary Fiber: Fiber that naturally occurs in plants. Fiber is classified as either soluble or insoluble in water.

Dried Sprouted Beans: A faster cooking and more easily digestible source of complex carbohydrates and protein as compared to unsprouted dried beans.

EPA (Eicosapentaenoic Acid): An essential, long-chain, polyunsaturated, omega-3 fatty acid. Food sources include herring, salmon, oysters and omega-3 enriched eggs.

Essential nutrient: A nutrient which must be obtained through diet; the body cannot synthesize required amounts necessary for health.

Folate: Needed for amino acid formation and DNA synthesis. Food sources include dark, leafy, green vegetables, beans and egg yolks.

Free radicals: A reactive molecule with one or more unpaired electron(s), potentially destructive to cell membranes, DNA and proteins.

Garam Masala: A warm spice blend used in Indian cuisine; frequently containing coriander seeds, cumin seeds, cardamom, black peppercorns, cinnamon and clove.

Glaucoma: A group of ocular maladies leading to optic nerve damage. Glaucoma is typically associated with an intraocular fluid pressure imbalance.

Glycemic Index: A rating system used to categorize foods based on their potential to effect the blood glucose response. Foods with higher glycemic index ratings raise blood sugar faster.

Glycemic Load: A rating system to categorize glycemic response, based upon the glycemic index and carbohydrate in a single serving.

Goji Berries (Wolfberries): A bright orange/red berry from a shrub native to China. They have high zinc and zeaxanthin concentrations.

Goldenberries (Cape Gooseberries): The mildly tart, goldenberry is closely related to tomatillos. Carotenoids give these berries their yellow-orange color. Dried goldenberries can be purchased at health food stores or online.

Iris: A thin, circular, pigmented structure located between the cornea and lens which constricts and dilates. This structure gives us our eye color.

LA (linoleic acid): An essential, polyunsaturated, omega-6 fatty acid, abundant in vegetable oils. Common food sources include safflower oil, grapeseed oil and corn oil.

Lens (crystalline lens): A transparent, biconvex structure made of protein responsible for focusing light onto the retina. A cloudy crystalline lens is known as a cataract.

Lutein: An essential carotenoid pigment found abundantly in the macula. Food sources of lutein include dark, leafy greens and yellow, fleshed fruit.

Lycopene: A fat-soluble carotenoid found abundantly in tomatoes. Cooking increases the bioavailability of lycopene.

Macronutrients: Nutrients required in larger quantities. These include proteins, carbohydrates and fats which provide our bodies with energy and structure.

Macula (macula lutea): A yellow, pigmented area at the center of retina responsible for sharp, detailed, central vision. The macula has a dense concentration of light-sensitive photoreceptors called cones.

Macular Degeneration: A deterioration of the central (macular) portion of the retina. The most common type of macular degeneration is known as Age-related Macular Degeneration (AMD).

Matcha: A high-quality, finely ground, green tea containing a potent group of antioxidants known as catechins.

Mexican Oregano: A culinary herb in the Verbena family that has a stronger, grassier flavor than Greek or Turkish oregano.

Micronutrients: Nutrients required in small quantities, such as the trace mineral zinc and organic compounds, such as vitamins.

Mineral: An inorganic substance required by the body in small quantities, such as zinc.

Mole: A sauce frequently used in Mexican cuisine containing dried peppers, chocolate and pepita seeds.

Nori (laver): A dried, edible seaweed used in sushi or crumbled as a seasoning. Nori is a good source of protein, fiber, Vitamins A, B, C, iron and zinc.

Nutrient synergy: Nutrients, when consumed together, enhance the effects of each other, more so than when eaten separately.

Omega-3 Eggs: Specialty eggs from chickens, pasture raised or fed oils rich in omega-3 fatty acids, such as krill oil, flax seed and algae oils. A good source of protein, omega-3 fatty acids, lutein+zeaxanthin, vitamin A, vitamin B complex, vitamin D and vitamin E.

Omega-3 fatty acids: A group of essential, polyunsaturated, fatty acids including: ALA found in plants; EPA and DHA commonly found in fish and some animal oils.

Omega-6 fatty acids: A group of essential polyunsaturated fatty acids found abundantly in vegetable oils, nuts, seeds and animal fats.

Optic disc (Optic nerve head): The structural area where retinal nerve fibers converge to form the optic nerve and where the central retinal blood supply enters and exits the eye. There are no photoreceptor cells on the optic disc and this creates what is known as the "blind spot" in our vision.

Optic nerve: The optic nerve contains bundled nerve fibers, originating from the photosensitive cells, rods and cones, to the brain.

Oregano: A culinary herb in the mint family; high in antioxidant activity from phenolic acid and flavonoids.

Pepita (Pumpkin) seeds: Frequently used in Mexican cuisine as a snack or a thickening agent in moles. A good source of protein, zinc and omega-3 fatty acids.

Phytonutrients: Biologically active compounds synthesized by plants with both foodlike and vitaminlike qualities.

Protein: A macronutrient composed of amino acids.

Pupil: The opening within the eye created by the constriction and dilation of the iris. A larger pupil allows more light to enter the eye and a smaller pupil limits the amount of light passing back to the retina.

Quinoa: An ancient, grain-like cereal from South America in the same food family as spinach, Swiss chard and beets. A quality, gluten-free source of the antioxidant flavonoids: quercetin and kaempferol. Rinse before using.

Retina: A neurological layer lining the inner eye containing the light-sensitive photoreceptor cells, rods and cones.

Rosewater: A floral-scented, distillate of rose petals frequently used in Middle-Eastern desserts.

Sclera: The opaque fibrous outer layer of the eye which is continuous with the transparent cornea, forming the eye ball.

Turbinado sugar: A raw, sugar-cane based, minimally refined sweetener with a high moisture content.

Vitamin A: A family of fat-soluble related compounds to include retinoids and the carotenoids.

Vitamin B: A group of distinct, water-soluble vitamins that often coexist in the same foods.

Vitamin B12 (Cobalamin): Involved in energy metabolism and production of blood cells in bone marrow, nerve sheaths and protein. Food sources include organ meat, fish and eggs.

Vitamin B6 (Pyroxidine): Integral to the metabolism of amino acids and lipids, and synthesis of neurotransmitters. Food sources include chicken, liver and tuna.

Vitamin C (Ascorbic Acid): A water-soluble, highly effective antioxidant used in the production of collagen. Food sources include red, bell pepper, broccoli and strawberries. Many tissues within the eye require high amounts of vitamin C.

Vitamin D: A group of fat-soluble, secosteroids responsible for the absorption of micronutrients within the body. Vitamin D can be ingested or it can be synthesized by the body with the aid of sunlight exposure.

Vitamin E: A family of eight fat soluble antioxidants, four tocopherols and four tocotrienols. Food sources include wheat germ oil, sunflower seeds and almonds.

Vitamin: An organic compound required in small amounts from the diet. Most vitamins cannot be synthesized in sufficient quantities by the body to promote good health.

Vitreous: A transparent, gelatinous mass inside the eye which helps to maintain the shape of the eye. It is located between the lens and retina and contains water, collagen, protein and hyaluronic acid.

Zeaxanthin: An essential phytochemical and carotenoid pigment found abundantly in the central macula. Zeaxanthin and lutein are frequently found together in food sources. Food source include goji berries, orange bell peppers and corn.

Zinc: An essential trace mineral involved in gene expression, immune function and cell growth. The retina has a high concentration of zinc. Food sources include oysters, beef and dark turkey meat.

SANDRA YOUNG, OD

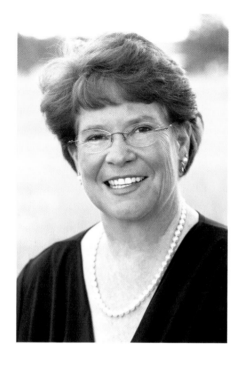

Sandra A. Young, OD is an optometrist with a special interest in nutrition and vision. She earned her Doctor of Optometry from Pacific University, College of Optometry, Forest Grove, Oregon, 1984. Dr. Young comes from a long line of chefs and waiters from New Orleans, both French and Italian. She has been cooking in the Mediterranean tradition since before the age of 10, both in her family's kitchen and catering for large events. After practicing optometry in private practice and military medical facilities, she began reviewing the compelling research in nutrition, vision and prevention of eye disease. She is inspired by current research to potentially curb through nutrition, the devastating vision impairing eye disease, macular degeneration she has seen in many elderly patients. This cookbook blends her exceptional cooking skills with her knowledge of current ocular science and research, creating a practical guide to ocular nutrition for her patients and the public at large. Dr. Young is convinced healthful meals the entire family will enjoy can be prepared with exceptional taste while supporting ocular health. She is married with two children. She is an avid golfer, enjoys playing tennis and family life.

ANNE MARIE COUTTS, DTR

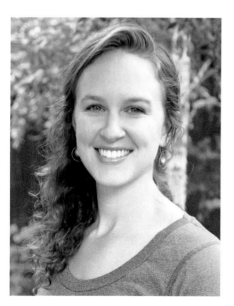

Anne Marie Coutts, DTR is a photographer and nutritional advisor. She received her bachelor's degree in nutrition from California Polytechnic State University in San Luis Obispo, 2011. During her studies she created healthful eating curricula for all ages, from children in Head Start Program Centers to patients with dementia in assisted living facilities. After graduation, she was Dietary Supervisor at San Fernando Post Acute Hospital in Southern California, where she earned her Dietetic Technician Registered (DTR) license by written and practical exam. Anne Marie developed a passion for photography early. She combined her expertise in photography with interests in food science, health, and wellness. Ultimately, her knowledge and talents in these areas all came together with the publication of this book. Anne Marie continues to innovatively style all types of culinary fare, capturing the images of these tasty dishes while providing maximum nutritional support with elegant simplicity. Besides photography and the culinary arts, she enjoys fitness, especially hiking and yoga.

References

Nutrition

Ames BN. Prevention of mutation, cancer, and other age-associated diseases by optimizing micronutrient intake. *J Nucleic Acids*. 2010 Sep 22; 2010

Ames BN. Optimal micronutrients delay mitochondrial decay and age-associated diseases. *Mech Ageing Dev*. 2010 Jul-Aug; 131(7-8): 473-9

Bian S, Gao Y, Zhang M, et al. Dietary nutrient intake and metabolic syndrome risk in Chinese adults: a case-control study. *Nutr J*. 2013 Jul 30; 12: 12-106 (a dietary B vitamin study)

Boeing H, Bechthoud Am Bub A, et al. Critical review: vegetables and fruit in the prevention of chronic diseases. *Eur J Nutr*. 2012 Sep; 51(6): 637-63

McCann JC, Ames BN. Is there convincing biological or behavioral evidence linking vitamin D deficiency to brain dysfunction? *FASEB J*. 2008 Apr; 22(4); 982-1001

McCann JC, Ames BN. Vitamin K, an example of triage theory: is micronutrient inadequacy linked to diseases of aging? *Am J Clin Nutr*. 2009 Oct; 90(4): 889-907

Sesso H, Buring J, Christen W, et al. Vitamins E and C in the Prevention of Cardiovascular Disease in Men - The Physicians' Health Study II Randomized Controlled Trial. *JAMA-Express*, Vol. 300 NO. 18. November 12, 2008

Vitamin C research funded by Arizona State University Foundation found that 3 percent of the incoming student population tested positive for scurvy. The National Health and Nutrition Examination Survey (NHANES III) reported 13 percent of US adult males and 9 percent of US adult females have blood vitamin C levels indicating scurvy. For more information, contact Carol Johnson, PhD, CNS, RD, at carol.johnston@asu.edu

Vitamins for chronic disease prevention in adults: scientific review. Fairfield KM, Fletcher RH. *JAMA*. 2002 Jun 19; 287(23):3116-26. Review.

Wilcox S, Sharpe PA, Turner-McGrievy G, Granner M, Baruth M. Frequency of consumption at fast-food restaurants is associated with dietary intake in overweight and obese women recruited from financially disadvantaged neighborhoods. *Nutr Res*. 2013 Aug; 33(8):636-46

AMD & Nutrition

Abu EJ-Asrar Am, Abdel Gader, AG, et al. Hyperhomocysteinemia and retinal vascular occlusive disease. Eur J Ophthalmology. 2002 Nov-Dec; 12(6):495-500

Age-Related Eye Disease Research Group. A randomized placebo-controlled clinical trial of high-dosed supplementation with vitamins C and E, beta carotene, and zinc for age-related macular degeneration and vision loss, AREDS Report No. 8. *Arch Ophthalmol*. 2001;119: 417-36.

Aydin E, Demir HD, et al. Association of plasma homocysteine and macular edema in type 2 diabetes mellitus. *Eur J Ophthalmol*. 2008 Mar-Apr; 18(2):226-32

Bian Q, Gao S, Zhou J et al. Lutein and zeaxanthin supplementation reduces photooxidative damage and modulates the expression of inflammation-related genes in retinal pigment epithelial cells. *Free Radic Biol Med*. 2012 Sep 15; 53(6); 1298-307

Christen W, Glynn R, Chew E, et al. Folic Acid, Pyridoxine, and Cyanocobalamin Combination Treatment and Age-Related Macular Degeneration in women. *Archives of Internal Medicine*. Vol 169 (4): Feb 23, 2009

Kijistra A, Tian Y, et al. Lutein: more than just a filter for blue light. *Prog Retin Eye Res*. 2012 Jul; 31(4): 303-15

Lutein + zeaxanthin and omega-3 fatty acids for age-related macular degeneration: the Age-Related Eye Disease Study 2 (AREDS2) randomized clinical trial. *JAMA*. 2013 May 15; 309(19): 2005-15

Seddon JM et al. Association between C-reactive protein and age-related macular degeneration. JAMA. 2004, 291: 704-10.

Tan JS. Wang JJ, et al. Dietary fatty acids and the 10-year incidence of age-related macular degeneration: the Blue Mountains Eye Study. *Arch Ophthalmol*. 2009 May; 127(5):656-65

Wilcox S, Sharpe PA, Turner-McGrievy G, Granner M, Baruth M. Frequency of consumption at fast-food restaurants is associated with dietary intake in overweight and obese women recruited from financially disadvantaged neighborhoods. *Nutr Res*. 2013 Aug; 33(8):636-46

Cataract & Nutrition

Chiu CJ, Milton RC, et al. Dietary carbohydrate intake and glycemic index in relation to cortical and nuclear lens opacities in the Age-Related Eye Disease Study. *Am J Clin Nutr*. 2006 May; 83(5):1177-84

Chiu CJ, Taylor A. Nutritional antioxidants and age-related cataract and maculopathy. Chiu CJ, Taylor A. *Exp Eye Res*. 2006 Jul 28

Fodrigues-Rodrigues E, Ortega RM el al. The relationship between antioxidant nutrient intake and cataracts in older people. *Int J Vitamin Nutr Res*. 2006 Nov; 76(6):359-66

Kisic B, Miric D, Zoric L, et al. Antioxidant capacity of lenses with age-related cataract. *Oxid Med Cell Longev*. 2012; 2012: 467130

Ravindran RD, Vashist P et al. Inverse association of vitamin C with cataract in older people in India. *Ophthalmology*. 2011 Oct; 118(10): 1958-1965

Tan J, Want JJ, Flood V, et al. Carbohydrate nutrition, glycemic index, and the 10 year incidence of cataract. *Am J Clin Nutr*. 2007 Nov; 86(5): 1502-8

Thiagrajan R, Manikandan R. Antioxidants and cataract. *Free Radic Res*. 2013 May; 47(5): 337-45

Glaucoma and Nutrition

Acar N, Berdeaux O, Juaneda P, et al. Red blood cell plasmalogens and docosahexaenoic acid are independently reduced in primary open-angle glaucoma. *Exp Eye Res*. 2009 Dec; 89(6): 840-53

Creuzot-Garcher C, Bron A. The place of micronutrition in glaucoma management. *J Fr Ophthalmol*. 2008 Jul; 31(6); 2S65-8

Evans SC. Ophthalmic nutrition and prevention of eye disorder and blindness. *Nutr Metab*. 1977; 21 Suppl 1: 268-72

Manze F. Hydration and disease. *J Am Coll Nutr*. 2007 Oct; 26(5): 535S-541S

Pasquale LR, Kang JH. Lifestyle, nutrition, and glaucoma. *J Glaucoma*. 2009 Aug; 18(6): 423-8

Ren H, Magulike N, et al. Primary open-angle glaucoma patients have reduced levels of blood docosahexaenoic and eicosapentaenoic acids. *Prostaglandins Leukot Essent Fatty Acids*. 2006 Mar; 74(3): 157-63

Veach J. Functional dichotomy: glutathione and vitamin E in homeostasis relevant to primary open-angle glaucoma. *Br J Nutr*. 2004 Jun; 91(6); 809-29

Inflammation & Nutrition

Block G, Jensen CD, Dalvi TB, Norkus EP, Hudes M, Crawford PB, Holland N, Fung EB, Schumacher L, Harmatz P Vitamin C treatment reduces elevated C-reactive protein. *Free Radic Biol Med*. 2008 Oct 10.

Ershler WB, Keller ET. Age-associated increased interleukin-6 gene expression, late-life diseases, and frailty. *Annu Rev Med*. 2000, 51:245-70.

Ford DE et al. Depression and C-reactive protein in US adults. *Arch Intern Med*. 2004, 164:1010-14.

Kop WJ et al. Inflammation and coagulation factors in persons > 65 years of age with symptoms of depression but without evidence of myocardial ischemia. *Am J Cardiol*. 2002, 89:419-24.

McGreer PL, McGreer EG. Inflammation and the degenerative diseases of aging. *Ann NY Acad Sci*. 2004, 1035:104-16.

Papanicolaou DA, et al. The pathophysiologic roles of interleukin-6 in human disease. *Ann Int Med*. 1998, 128:127-37.

Schmidt R et al. Early inflammation and dementia: a 25-year follow-up of the Honolulu-Asia Aging Study. *Ann Neurol.* 2002, 52:168-74.

Dementia & Nutrition

Bhullar KS, Rupasinghe HP. Polyphenols: multipotent therapeutic agents in neurodegenerative diseases. *Oxid Med Cell Longev.* 2013; 2013: 8917

Chin D, Huebbe P, et al. Neuroprotective Properties of Curcumin in Alzheimer's disease – Merits and Limitations. *Curr Med Chem.* 2013 Aug 6

Droogsma E, van Asselt DZ, Scholzel-Dorenbos CJ. Et al. Nutritional status of community-dwelling elderly with newly diagnosed Alzheimer's disease: prevalence of malnutrition and the relation of various factors to nutritional status. *J Nutr Health Aging.* 2013; 17(7): 606-10

Hu N, Yu JT, Tan L, et al. Nutrition and the risk of Alzheimer's disease. *Biomed Res Int.* 2013; 2013: 524820

Otaegui-Arrazola A, Amiano P, Elbusto A, Urdaneta E, Martinex-Lag P. Diet, cognition, and Alzheimer's disease: food for thought. *Eur J Nutr.* 2014 Jul 27

Schmidt R et al. Early inflammation and dementia: a 25-year follow-up of the Honolulu-Asia Aging Study. Ann Neurol. 2002, 52:168-74.

Type II Diabetes & Nutrition

Blondin SA, Yeung EH, Mumford SL et al. Serum Retinol and Carotenoids in Association with Biomarkers of Insulin Resistance among Premenopausal Women. *ISRN Nutr.* 2013 Jan 1; 2013: 619516

Festa A et al. Chronic subclinical inflammation as part of the insulin resistance syndrome. *Circ* 2000. 102: 42-47.

Higher dietary flavonol intake is associated with lower incidence of type 2 diabetes. *J Nutr.* 2013 Jul 31

Lee Y-H, Pratley RE. The evolving role of inflammation in obesity and the metabolic syndrome. *Curr Diab Rep.* 2005, 5:70-75.

Pedersen AN, Kondrup J, Bersheim E. Health effects of protein intake in healthy adults: a systematic literature review. *Food Nutr Res.* 2014 Jul 30: 57

Pradhan AD et al. C-reactive protein, interleukin-6, and risk of developing type 2 diabetes. *JAMA.* 2001, 286:327-34.

Sarboluki S, Javanbakht MH, et al. Eicosapentaenoic acid improves insulin sensitivity and blood sugar in overweight type 2 diabetes mellitus patients: a double-blind randomized clinical trial. *Singapore Med J.* 2013 Jul; 54 (7): 387-90.

Xu H et al. Chronic inflammation in fat plays a crucial role in the development of obesity-related insulin resistance. *J Clin Invest.* 2003, 112: 1821-30.

Resources

About Nutrition
http://www.nutrition.about.com

Environmental Working Group
http://www.ewg.org

Linus Pauling Institute at Oregon State University. Micronutrient Research for Optimal Health. www.lpi.oregonstate.edu/infocenter

Ocular Nutrition Society
http://www.ocularnutritionsociety.org

Self Nutrition Data
http://www.nutritiondata.self.com

United States Department of Agriculture Nutrient Data Base. National Agricultural Library. www.fnic.nal.usda.gov/food-composition

World's Healthiest Foods
http://www.whfoods.com

Nutritional Content of Achiote/Annatto Seeds

Upon review of the literature, annatto seeds contain both vitamin E tocotrienols and carotenoids, however the amount per serving was indeterminate. This represents an opportunity for further research into nutrition and vision.

VISIONARY KITCHEN
SHOPPING LIST

Vegetables & Fresh Herbs

☐ _____
☐ _____
☐ _____
☐ _____
☐ _____
☐ _____

Fruit

☐ _____
☐ _____
☐ _____
☐ _____
☐ _____
☐ _____

Fish & Shellfish

☐ _____
☐ _____
☐ _____
☐ _____

Poultry & Lean Meat

☐ _____
☐ _____
☐ _____
☐ _____

Nuts & Seeds

☐ _____
☐ _____
☐ _____
☐ _____

Dairy, Eggs & Tofu

☐ _____
☐ _____
☐ _____
☐ _____

Grains, Beans & Legumes

☐ _____
☐ _____
☐ _____

Dried Herbs & Spices

☐ _____
☐ _____
☐ _____

Superfood Eye Treats

☐ _____
☐ _____
☐ _____

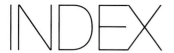

INDEX

Special Diets, listed by recipe title:
- Ⓥ vegetarian
- Ⓔ vegan
- Ⓓ dairy-free
- Ⓖ gluten-free